Neuromuscular Diseases - How to Recognize and Treat Them

Edited by Simona Maria Carmignano

Published in London, United Kingdom

Neuromuscular Diseases - How to Recognize and Treat Them
http://dx.doi.org/10.5772/intechopen.1004494
Edited by Simona Maria Carmignano

Contributors
Adamantios Katerelos, Alessandra Carneiro Dorça, Chee Shin Yong, Fatemeh Mansouri, Fatima Rawas, Hassan Doumiati, Hideki Nakano, Kamala Oghuz, Kotaro Nakagawa, Letícia de Araújo Morais, Maede Makhtoomi, Maria Clotilde Tavares, Marzieh Mahmoodi, Mathew Alexander, Mehran Nouri, Naoki Shimizu, Ryosuke Yamamoto, Shoya Fujikawa, Shun Sawai, Simona Maria Carmignano, Valeska Kouzak, Wendy Isabel Silvestre da Silva, Yusuke Shizuka, Zainab Shateri

First published in London, United Kingdom, 2025 by IntechOpen
IntechOpen is the global imprint of INTECHOPEN LIMITED, registered in England and Wales, registration number: 11086078, 167-169 Great Portland Street, London, W1W 5PF, United Kingdom

For EU product safety concerns: IN TECH d.o.o., Prolaz Marije Krucifikse Kozulić 3, 51000 Rijeka, Croatia, info@intechopen.com or visit our website at intechopen.com.

British Library Cataloguing-in-Publication Data
A catalogue record for this book is available from the British Library

Neuromuscular Diseases - How to Recognize and Treat Them
Edited by Simona Maria Carmignano
p. cm.
Print ISBN 978-1-83634-254-0
Online ISBN 978-1-83634-253-3
eBook (PDF) ISBN 978-1-83634-255-7

Meet the editor

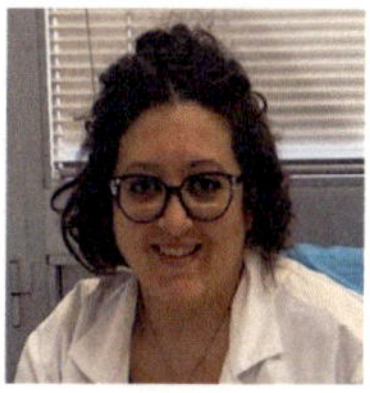

Simona Maria Carmignano is an Italian specialist in Physical and Rehabilitation Medicine. Born on June 5, 1984, she graduated with honours in Medicine and Surgery from the University of Chieti in 2012. Subsequently, she specialized in Physical and Rehabilitation Medicine in 2017. Dr. Carmignano currently works as a consultant physician at the CTR Therapeutic Rehabilitation Center in Tramutola and serves as a contract professor at the University of Salerno. Her expertise focuses on innovative rehabilitation techniques, significantly contributing to treating Parkinson's disease, stroke recovery, and gait training using robotics. She has authored numerous scientific publications and book chapters in her field, underscoring her dedication to advancing rehabilitation medicine.

Contents

Preface

Neuromuscular diseases encompass a wide range of disorders that affect both the nervous system and muscles, often profoundly impacting a patient's quality of life. Despite the significant strides made in medicine and research, many of these conditions are still diagnosed late, which can complicate treatment and limit the potential for improvement. In this context, it becomes increasingly important for healthcare providers to understand how to recognize and treat these diseases in order to offer the best care possible.

Neuromuscular Diseases – How to Recognize and Treat Them aims to fill this gap by providing a thorough and accessible guide to the most common neuromuscular disorders. The goal of this book is simple yet crucial: to give healthcare professionals the knowledge and tools they need to make timely diagnoses and provide the most effective treatments. The author takes a thoughtful and clear approach, breaking down complex medical concepts while maintaining scientific accuracy.

Throughout the chapters, you'll find an exploration of the key aspects of neuromuscular diseases, from the underlying biology and symptoms to the latest advancements in treatment options. Clinical cases and real-life examples provide practical insights, helping the reader better understand how these diseases present and how to approach their management.

As the medical field continues to evolve, it's vital for those in healthcare to stay updated on new diagnostic and treatment techniques. This book provides a solid foundation of knowledge and invites reflection on how we can improve our daily clinical practices, tailor treatments to individual patients, and foster collaboration across specialties.

I hope you find this book informative and thought-provoking and that it serves as a valuable tool for navigating the complexities of neuromuscular diseases. I hope it will help increase awareness and improve care for those living with these challenging conditions.

Simona Maria Carmignano
CTR Rehabilitation Therapy Center,
Basilicata, Tramutola, Italy

Adjunct Professor,
DIPMED, University of Salerno,
Italy

Section 1

Neuromuscular Diseases and Risk Factors

Chapter 1

Genetic Neuromuscular Diseases

Adamantios Katerelos

Abstract

Genetic neuromuscular diseases are a diverse group of disorders caused by mutations that impact muscle fibers, motor neurons, and neuromuscular junctions. Notable examples of these disorders include Duchenne muscular dystrophy (DMD), spinal muscular atrophy (SMA), and myotonic dystrophy, all of which manifest symptoms such as progressive muscle weakness and atrophy. Recent advancements in genetic diagnostics, particularly whole-exome sequencing, have significantly enhanced the accuracy of diagnoses and facilitated the development of personalized treatment strategies, which are crucial for improving patient outcomes. Innovative therapeutic approaches, such as gene therapy and CRISPR-Cas9 technology, hold considerable potential for rectifying genetic anomalies and creating targeted treatment options. Current research endeavors aim to expand our comprehension of the underlying mechanisms of these disorders, with particular emphasis on inflammation and cellular repair mechanisms. As our understanding evolves, there is optimism for the emergence of more effective therapeutic interventions, ultimately leading to an improved quality of life for individuals affected by these complex conditions.

Keywords: genetic neuromuscular disorder, muscular dystrophy, myopathy, genetic testing, neurological disorder

1. Introduction

Genetic neuromuscular diseases encompass a diverse group of conditions with underlying genetic etiologies [1]. These disorders, such as muscular dystrophies, myopathies, and myasthenic syndromes, are primarily inherited and can manifest with a wide range of clinical presentations [2]. The genetic landscape of neuromuscular diseases is complex, with variations in inheritance patterns including autosomal recessive, dominant, or X-linked modes [2]. Advances in genetic testing, particularly through techniques like next-generation sequencing (NGS) and exome sequencing, have significantly enhanced the diagnostic capabilities for these conditions [3]. These technologies have enabled a more comprehensive understanding of the genetic basis of neuromuscular disorders, leading to improved genotype–phenotype correlations [3].

The genetic heterogeneity of neuromuscular diseases poses challenges in diagnosis and management [4]. Conditions like congenital myasthenic syndromes (CMS) exemplify this complexity, with mutations affecting proteins crucial for neuromuscular junction function [5]. The identification of causative genes for these disorders has expanded over the years, shedding light on the molecular mechanisms underlying these conditions [6]. Furthermore, the overlap in clinical presentations among different neuromuscular disorders underscores the importance of genetic testing in providing accurate diagnoses [4].

Genetic testing plays a pivotal role in the management of neuromuscular disorders, offering benefits such as less invasiveness, cost-effectiveness, and timely diagnosis [7]. The American Association of Neuromuscular and Electrodiagnostic Medicine (AANEM) recognizes the significance of genetic testing in these conditions, emphasizing its role in diagnosis, disease management, and family planning [8]. Additionally, genetic studies have revealed that approximately 25% of genes associated with cardiomyopathy also contribute to neuromuscular disorders, highlighting the interconnectedness of these conditions at a genetic level [9].

The advent of next-generation sequencing has revolutionized the evaluation of genetically heterogeneous neuromuscular disorders [10]. These technologies have significantly improved the diagnostic yield, with studies reporting definitive molecular diagnoses in a substantial percentage of cases [11]. Despite the challenges posed by the clinical and genetic heterogeneity of these disorders, genetic testing has emerged as a valuable tool in elucidating their underlying genetic causes [4].

In the realm of genetic therapies, advancements in genome editing techniques offer promising avenues for the treatment of inherited neuromuscular diseases [12]. These approaches target a broad spectrum of genetic mutations, including point mutations, insertions, deletions, and chromosomal rearrangements, with the potential to address the root genetic causes of these conditions [13]. Moreover, the utilization of CRISPR-based gene therapies holds great potential for addressing the genetic underpinnings of neuromuscular disorders, albeit with distinct challenges in clinical translation [12].

2. Genetics and inheritance patterns

Genetic neuromuscular diseases encompass a variety of inheritance patterns, showcasing the genetic complexity inherent in these conditions. For example, myotonic dystrophy type 1 and Limb–Girdle muscular dystrophy Type 2B (LGMD2B) illustrate the diverse genetic landscape of neuromuscular disorders, with LGMD2B following an autosomal recessive pattern of inheritance Hauschild [14]. Understanding these specific inheritance patterns is crucial for precise diagnosis and genetic counseling. Moreover, the co-occurrence of myotonic dystrophy and LGMD highlights the intricate genetic interactions contributing to these conditions.

In the realm of prenatal diagnosis and genetic testing for neuromuscular diseases, next-generation sequencing (NGS) has emerged as a powerful tool [3]. NGS and exome sequencing have transformed genetic diagnostics, enhancing the understanding of genotype–phenotype correlations in neuromuscular diseases. These technologies have significantly improved the identification of causative genetic variants in patients with neuromuscular disorders, aiding in early diagnosis and intervention.

The inheritance patterns of genetic neuromuscular diseases can exhibit unique characteristics based on parental transmission. For instance, in myotonic dystrophy type 1, the age of onset of signs and symptoms can vary depending on whether the disease is inherited from the mother or the father [15]. This underscores the impact of parental inheritance on disease presentation and emphasizes the importance of considering the specific genetic mechanisms involved in each case.

Digenic inheritance, as observed in dysferlinopathy, challenges traditional models of recessive inheritance by revealing the complex interplay of multiple genetic factors in disease manifestation [16]. Understanding such atypical inheritance patterns is essential for unraveling the genetic basis of neuromuscular disorders and emphasizes the necessity of comprehensive genetic testing approaches to capture the full spectrum of genetic variations contributing to these conditions.

The prevalence of neuromuscular diseases can vary among populations, as demonstrated by studies in regions such as Southern China and Thailand [17, 18]. These variations underscore the influence of genetic and environmental factors on the prevalence of inherited neuromuscular disorders. Additionally, exploring the genetic spectrum of neuromuscular disorders in different populations, including Africans, is crucial to elucidate the unique genetic landscape of these conditions [19].

Advancements in next-generation sequencing technologies have significantly enhanced the molecular diagnosis of genetically inherited neuromuscular disorders [20]. These technologies enable rapid and comprehensive molecular diagnosis, aiding in the identification of disease-causing genetic variants in patients with neuromuscular conditions. The evolving landscape of genetic testing plays a vital role in unraveling the genetic complexity of neuromuscular diseases and guiding personalized treatment strategies.

The genetic underpinnings of neuromuscular diseases often extend beyond the muscular system, impacting other organ systems such as the cardiovascular system. Inherited neuromuscular disorders can be associated with hypertrophic cardiomyopathy, emphasizing the systemic nature of these conditions [21]. Understanding the genetic links between neuromuscular and cardiovascular manifestations is essential for comprehensive patient care and highlights the importance of multidisciplinary management approaches.

The genetics and inheritance patterns of genetic neuromuscular diseases are multifaceted, encompassing a spectrum of inheritance modes ranging from autosomal recessive and dominant patterns to digenic inheritance. Advances in genetic testing technologies, such as next-generation sequencing, have revolutionized the diagnosis and understanding of these conditions. By unraveling the genetic complexities of neuromuscular disorders and exploring diverse inheritance patterns, researchers and clinicians can pave the way for more precise diagnostics, personalized treatment strategies, and improved outcomes for individuals affected by these conditions.

3. Common types of genetic neuromuscular diseases

The prevalent categories of genetic neuromuscular disorders include a diverse range of conditions that impact the neuromuscular system as a result of genetic influences. Duchenne muscular dystrophy (DMD) stands out as one of the most prevalent and well-known genetic neuromuscular diseases, characterized by progressive muscle weakness and degeneration Chen [22]. This condition, caused by mutations in the DMD gene, leads to the absence of dystrophin, a protein crucial for muscle function. Another common type is spinal muscular atrophy (SMA), a genetic disorder affecting motor neurons in the spinal cord, resulting in muscle weakness and atrophy [23]. SMA is caused by deletions or mutations in the SMN1 gene, impacting the production of survival motor neuron (SMN) protein essential for motor neuron function.

Myotonic dystrophy type 1 (DM1) is another prevalent genetic neuromuscular disease characterized by muscle weakness, myotonia, and multi-systemic involvement

[24]. DM1 is caused by an expansion of CTG repeats in the DMPK gene, leading to the production of toxic RNA molecules that disrupt cellular functions. Additionally, Charcot–Marie–Tooth disease (CMT) represents a group of inherited peripheral neuropathies affecting motor and sensory nerves, leading to muscle weakness and sensory loss [25]. CMT encompasses various subtypes, each associated with distinct genetic mutations affecting peripheral nerve function.

Congenital myasthenic syndromes (CMS) constitute a group of genetic neuromuscular disorders characterized by impaired neuromuscular transmission, resulting in muscle weakness and fatigue [26]. These syndromes involve mutations in genes encoding proteins critical for neuromuscular junction function. Furthermore, Limb–Girdle muscular dystrophy (LGMD) encompasses a group of genetic disorders characterized by progressive muscle weakness predominantly affecting the shoulder and hip girdle muscles [27]. LGMD comprises multiple subtypes, each associated with specific genetic mutations impacting muscle structure and function.

Facioscapulohumeral muscular dystrophy (FSHD) is a genetic neuromuscular disease characterized by progressive muscle weakness, particularly in the face, shoulders, and upper arms. FSHD is linked to the deletion of repetitive DNA sequences near the DUX4 gene, leading to abnormal gene expression and muscle degeneration [28]. Additionally, myasthenia gravis (MG) represents an autoimmune neuromuscular disorder characterized by muscle weakness and fatigue due to autoantibodies targeting the neuromuscular junction. MG can have genetic predispositions and is often associated with specific HLA gene variants [29].

In summary, common types of genetic neuromuscular diseases encompass a spectrum of conditions affecting the neuromuscular system due to underlying genetic mutations. These disorders, such as Duchenne muscular dystrophy, spinal muscular atrophy, myotonic dystrophy type 1, Charcot–Marie–Tooth disease, congenital myasthenic syndromes, Limb–Girdle muscular dystrophy, facioscapulohumeral muscular dystrophy, and myasthenia gravis, highlight the diverse genetic landscape of neuromuscular disorders and underscore the importance of genetic testing and personalized management strategies in these conditions.

4. Clinical presentation and symptoms

The clinical features and symptoms associated with genetic neuromuscular diseases exhibit a wide range of manifestations, which can differ based on the particular disorder involved. Myasthenia gravis (MG), for instance, may exhibit worsening symptoms influenced by factors such as emotional distress, systemic diseases like viral respiratory infections, and certain medications affecting neuromuscular transmission [30]. In Duchenne muscular dystrophy (DMD), profound hyperCKemia can be observed, along with muscle weakness and degeneration, highlighting the importance of early diagnosis through next-generation sequencing and chromosomal microarray analysis [31].

Oculopharyngeal muscular dystrophy (OPMD) presents clinical features that overlap with other neuromuscular diseases, making diagnosis challenging. These features may resemble conditions like myasthenia gravis, Kearns–Sayre syndrome, and inclusion body myositis (IBM), emphasizing the need for precise diagnostic methods such as insoluble poly-A binding protein nuclear 1 (PABPN1) accumulation assessment [32]. Muscle magnetic resonance imaging (MRI) of the lower limbs serves as a valuable diagnostic tool in childhood neuromuscular disorders, aiding in the identification of characteristic findings in various neuromuscular conditions [33].

Whole exome sequencing has proven to be diagnostically useful in the neuromuscular clinic, with targeted single gene testing remaining a common diagnostic approach for many patients [34]. In the case of congenital LMNA (lamin A/C)-related muscular dystrophy, personalized cardiac management strategies have been implemented to prevent malignant arrhythmias in affected individuals [35]. Additionally, chronic spinal muscular atrophy (SMA) prognosis is significantly influenced by patient age, impacting disease duration and neuromuscular damage progression [36].

Exome sequencing in pediatric neuromuscular clinics has led to more frequent diagnoses of both neuromuscular and neurodevelopmental conditions, highlighting the importance of comprehensive genetic testing approaches [37]. The prevalence of inherited neuromuscular diseases can vary among populations, as evidenced by studies in regions like Southern China, emphasizing the influence of genetic and environmental factors on disease prevalence [17]. Furthermore, the genetic spectrum of cardiomyopathies with a neuromuscular phenotype underscores the interconnectedness of cardiac and neuromuscular manifestations in certain genetic conditions [38].

Facioscapulohumeral muscular dystrophy (FSHD) typically presents with symptoms beginning in childhood, with over 90% of patients showing signs of the disease by age 20 [28, 39]. Autoimmune inflammatory myopathies share common pathways with genetic neuromuscular disorders, suggesting potential overlapping mechanisms in disease pathogenesis [40]. Prenatal ultrasonic presentations in fetuses with monogenic neurologic and neuromuscular diseases can provide important clues for prenatal diagnosis, particularly through the identification of abnormal fetal gestures and movements [41].

In summary, the clinical manifestations and symptoms associated with genetic neuromuscular disorders exhibit considerable diversity and complexity, encompassing a spectrum that includes muscle weakness and atrophy, as well as cardiac issues and respiratory difficulties. Advances in genetic testing technologies, such as exome sequencing and chromosomal microarray analysis, have significantly improved diagnostic capabilities, enabling early identification and personalized management strategies for individuals affected by these conditions. Understanding the nuanced clinical features and genetic underpinnings of neuromuscular diseases is essential for accurate diagnosis, prognosis, and treatment planning.

5. Management and treatment strategies

The strategies for managing and treating genetic neuromuscular disorders require a multidisciplinary approach, designed to tackle the varied clinical presentations and genetic intricacies associated with these diseases. Therapies targeting the neonatal Fc receptor (FcRn) have emerged as a promising strategy for managing autoantibody-mediated diseases by modulating IgG recycling and facilitating immunomodulation Jaffry [42]. Additionally, the conservation of selective vulnerability in amyotrophic lateral sclerosis and spinal muscular atrophy highlights the potential for developing therapeutic interventions to protect the vulnerable neuromuscular system [43].

Prior to discussing treatment options, it is essential to address the significance of functional rehabilitation for individuals diagnosed with JALS. This rehabilitation employs a multidisciplinary strategy aimed at optimizing independence, functionality, and overall quality of life. Given the progressive characteristics of ALS, supportive therapies play a vital role in alleviating symptoms and enhancing the patient's holistic well-being.

Physical therapy is a fundamental component in addressing muscle weakness and spasticity that accompany juvenile ALS. Key interventions encompass stretching and range-of-motion exercises, which are instrumental in mitigating spasticity and enhancing mobility—an essential aspect as muscle function deteriorates. Additionally, strengthening exercises can be advantageous for muscles that retain some strength, and these should be customized according to the individual's capabilities and the progression of the disease. Implementing energy conservation techniques is also critical; patients learn strategies to execute daily tasks more effectively, thereby extending their functional abilities. The prompt introduction of assistive devices, such as lightweight ankle–foot orthoses, can significantly reduce the risk of falls and enhance mobility [44].

Occupational therapy aims to empower patients to sustain their daily living skills while adapting to their evolving physical limitations. This may involve recommending adaptive tools that facilitate everyday tasks, thereby promoting independence, or suggesting modifications to the home environment to enhance accessibility and safety [45, 46].

As ALS advances, patients frequently experience challenges with communication and swallowing. Speech therapy may encompass techniques designed to improve speech clarity and alternative communication methods, such as communication boards or electronic devices, particularly for those with bulbar involvement. Additionally, assessments and adjustments to dietary consistency are crucial to prevent aspiration and ensure safe swallowing [45, 46].

Furthermore, mental health support is imperative for both patients and their families. Therapeutic interventions can effectively address the emotional and psychological ramifications of living with this condition [45, 46].

In concluding the discussion on relief strategies for patients with JALS, it is essential to highlight the significant role of emerging technologies in enhancing patient support and comfort. The management of mobility for these individuals has increasingly integrated advanced technologies, robotics, and orthotic devices. These innovations are designed to improve mobility, foster independence, and elevate the overall quality of life for those grappling with the progressive challenges posed by this neurodegenerative condition.

Telemedicine has emerged as an indispensable resource for managing ALS, particularly in light of the COVID-19 pandemic. It facilitates remote monitoring of critical health indicators, such as respiratory function and nutritional status, thereby minimizing the necessity for in-person consultations, which can be particularly burdensome for patients with mobility constraints [47, 48].

Furthermore, brain–computer interfaces (BCI) and eye tracking technologies have broadened the avenues for communication and interaction for ALS patients. These systems empower individuals to operate devices and communicate through eye movements, which is especially advantageous as muscular control wanes. Such technologies not only enhance communication capabilities but also hold promise for managing mobility aids and smart home systems [47, 48].

The exploration of robotic devices for mobility assistance and rehabilitation is ongoing. These devices range from robotic exoskeletons that facilitate walking to robotic arms that support daily tasks. Although these technologies are primarily found in research environments at present, they offer significant potential for improving mobility and independence among ALS patients [47, 49].

Orthotic devices are also crucial in aiding mobility for individuals with ALS. Ankle–foot orthoses (AFOs), for instance, can stabilize the ankle and foot, thereby enhancing gait and minimizing fall risks. Additionally, customized wheelchairs and powered mobility devices can provide greater autonomy for patients as their mobility declines [46, 48].

Assistive technologies (AT) hold equal significance. AT refer to a diverse array of devices aimed at facilitating daily living tasks. For individuals with ALS, such technologies may consist of adaptive utensils and eating aids that are specifically engineered to assist with feeding as manual dexterity diminishes, as well as communication devices that employ speech-generating technology to enable effective communication as verbal abilities wane [46, 48].

Transitioning to the domain of science, we now turn our attention to the role of genetics. Genetic testing, particularly through next-generation sequencing technologies, plays a pivotal role in diagnosing and managing neuromuscular diseases. Studies have shown that unbiased genomic approaches, such as whole exome sequencing, can serve as powerful diagnostic tools for conditions with high clinical and genetic heterogeneity, enabling personalized treatment strategies [50]. Furthermore, the restoration of ubiquitin-like modifier activating enzyme 1(UBA1) has been demonstrated to ameliorate disease progression in spinal muscular atrophy, emphasizing the potential of targeting ubiquitin pathway defects for developing novel therapeutic approaches [51].

Artificial intelligence applications in diagnosing neuromuscular diseases offer innovative avenues for enhancing diagnostic accuracy and efficiency. Modeling neuromuscular tissues on a chip using advanced technologies has the potential to capture the diverse genotypes and phenotypes of individuals with various neuromuscular disorders, paving the way for personalized therapeutic approaches [52]. Moreover, the optimization of targeted exome sequencing has been identified as a sensitive and cost-effective method for diagnosing genetic neuromuscular disorders [53].

Immunosuppressive and immunomodulatory therapies have significantly impacted the treatment of immune-mediated neuromuscular diseases, highlighting the importance of tailored therapeutic approaches [54]. Antisense oligonucleotides (AONs) have shown promise in correcting genetic diseases through exon skipping, with the potential to address a wide range of neuromuscular disorders [55]. Additionally, gene therapy and genome editing technologies offer novel avenues for treating genetic neuromuscular diseases by targeting specific genetic mutations and pathways [13].

The clinical and genetic heterogeneity of neuromuscular diseases underscores the need for personalized therapeutic strategies. Advances in precision medicine have paved the way for tailored treatment approaches that consider individual genetic profiles and disease characteristics [56]. The development of novel therapies, such as exon skipping and gene replacement therapy, has revolutionized the management of neuromuscular diseases, offering hope for improved outcomes and quality of life for affected individuals [57].

In summary, the effective management and treatment of genetic neuromuscular disorders necessitate a holistic strategy that encompasses targeted palliative and therapeutic interventions, immunomodulatory treatments, genetic testing, and the application of cutting-edge technologies. By leveraging advancements in precision medicine, gene therapy, and artificial intelligence, clinicians can tailor treatment strategies to individual patients, addressing the complex genetic and clinical aspects of neuromuscular disorders. The evolving landscape of therapeutic interventions holds promise for improving outcomes and quality of life for individuals affected by genetic neuromuscular diseases.

6. Research and future directions

The field of genetic neuromuscular diseases (NMDs) is rapidly evolving, driven by advancements in genetic testing, novel therapeutic approaches, and a growing understanding of the underlying molecular mechanisms. Future directions in this area are focused on enhancing diagnostic accuracy, developing targeted therapies, and improving patient care through personalized medicine. This synthesis discusses these key areas, supported by relevant literature.

One of the most significant advancements in the diagnosis of genetic neuromuscular diseases is the application of next-generation sequencing (NGS). NGS has revolutionized the diagnostic process by allowing for comprehensive genetic testing that can identify a wide range of mutations associated with various neuromuscular disorders. For instance, the use of targeted gene panels has been shown to increase diagnostic yields significantly, providing critical information for patient management and treatment options [8, 10]. As the technology continues to improve, it is expected that the diagnostic capabilities will expand further, allowing for the identification of previously unrecognized genetic variants and phenotypes [34, 37].

In addition to NGS, the integration of multiomics approaches—combining genomics, transcriptomics, proteomics, and metabolomics—holds great promise for advancing our understanding of neuromuscular diseases. These approaches can elucidate the complex interactions between genetic factors and disease phenotypes, potentially leading to the identification of novel therapeutic targets [58]. For example, the application of machine learning algorithms to analyze multiomics data may enhance the accuracy of genetic diagnoses and improve patient stratification for clinical trials [59].

The development of gene therapies represents another exciting avenue for the treatment of genetic neuromuscular disorders. Recent advancements in gene therapy, particularly for conditions such as spinal muscular atrophy (SMA) and Duchenne muscular dystrophy (DMD), have demonstrated the potential to significantly modify disease progression [60, 61]. The approval of gene therapies targeting specific genetic mutations has opened new possibilities for treatment, but ongoing research is needed to assess the long-term safety and efficacy of these interventions [62]. Furthermore, efforts to expand gene therapy applications to older patients and those with pre-existing conditions are underway, highlighting the need for continued innovation in this area [63].

The use of patient-derived stem cells for modeling genetic neuromuscular diseases is another promising direction. These models enable researchers to study disease mechanisms in vitro and test potential therapeutic interventions in a controlled environment [64, 65]. The ability to generate high-throughput, automated tissue-engineered models will facilitate preclinical and clinical applications, accelerating the development of effective therapies 23. Additionally, the exploration of optogenetic techniques to quantify neuromuscular function may provide insights into disease mechanisms and therapeutic responses [64].

Despite these advancements, disparities in healthcare access and genetic testing remain a significant challenge, particularly in low- and middle-income countries. The need for improved genetic diagnostic capabilities and healthcare resources is critical to address the burden of neuromuscular diseases in underserved populations [19]. Initiatives such as the International Centre for Genomic Medicine in Neuromuscular Diseases aim to bridge these gaps by providing resources and support for genetic testing and research in these regions [19, 66].

Moreover, the psychosocial aspects of living with genetic neuromuscular disorders must not be overlooked. The emotional and psychological impact of these diseases on patients and their families can be profound, necessitating a holistic approach that includes mental health support alongside medical treatment [67]. The development of patient registries and natural history studies will be crucial for understanding the long-term outcomes of genetic therapies and improving care strategies for individuals with NMDs [68, 69].

In conclusion, the future of genetic neuromuscular diseases is promising, characterized by rapid advancements in genetic testing, innovative therapeutic approaches, and a growing understanding of disease mechanisms. Continued research and collaboration among clinicians, researchers, and patients will be essential to translate these advancements into improved diagnostic and therapeutic strategies, ultimately enhancing the quality of life for individuals affected by these complex disorders.

7. Conclusion

Genetic neuromuscular disorders represent a multifaceted and varied array of conditions that pose considerable difficulties in both diagnosis and treatment. A collaborative strategy that includes neurologists, physical therapists, occupational therapists, speech therapists, and mental health specialists is essential at the outset. This multidisciplinary team engages in ongoing assessment and modification of rehabilitation plans to align with the patient's changing requirements. It is crucial to regularly reassess and modify treatment approaches to effectively meet the intricate and dynamic needs of patients. The integration of advanced technologies, robotics, and orthotic devices in the treatment of juvenile ALS patients marks a significant advancement in enhancing mobility and overall quality of life. These technological innovations not only facilitate physical movement but also empower patients to sustain communication and autonomy, which are vital for individuals coping with a progressive illness such as ALS. Ongoing innovation and implementation of these technologies will be imperative to tackle the specific challenges encountered by this demographic.

Recent progress in genetic diagnostics, particularly through the implementation of next-generation sequencing (NGS) and exome sequencing, has markedly enhanced the ability to diagnose these disorders, facilitating personalized treatment approaches and refining genotype–phenotype correlations. The genetic framework of neuromuscular diseases is distinguished by various inheritance patterns, including autosomal recessive, dominant, and X-linked inheritance, each presenting distinct challenges in comprehending and managing these intricate conditions. The introduction of next-generation sequencing has transformed the assessment of genetically diverse neuromuscular disorders, significantly increasing diagnostic success rates and assisting in the discovery of genetic variants responsible for the diseases. Additionally, the emergence of novel therapeutic strategies, such as gene therapy and CRISPR-Cas9 technology, presents promising opportunities for treating inherited neuromuscular disorders, highlighting the potential for targeted interventions to correct genetic defects. The outlook for genetic neuromuscular diseases is optimistic, characterized by swift advancements in genetic testing, pioneering therapeutic methods, and an expanding understanding of disease mechanisms. Ongoing research initiatives and collaboration among healthcare professionals, researchers, and patients will be crucial in converting these advancements into enhanced diagnostic and treatment strategies, ultimately improving the quality of life for those affected by these complex conditions.

Acknowledgement

The author acknowledges the use of InstaText (AI tool) for language polishing (to improve clarity, style, and readability in the document) of the manuscript.

Author details

Adamantios Katerelos
Neurology Department, Karamandaneio Children's Hospital, Patras, Greece

*Address all correspondence to: ad_katerelos@yahoo.gr

References

[1] Marchant R. Genome and rna sequencing boost neuromuscular diagnoses to 62% from 34% with exome sequencing alone. Annals of Clinical and Translational Neurology. 2024;**11**(5):1250-1266. DOI: 10.1002/acn3.52041

[2] Eshrif S. Profile of neuromuscular disorders: Neurology clinic, tripoli children hospital. Ibnosina Journal of Medicine and Biomedical Sciences. 2023;**15**(04):168-172. DOI: 10.1055/s-0043-1772820

[3] Todd E, Yau K, Ong R, Slee J, McGillivray G, Barnett C, et al. Next generation sequencing in a large cohort of patients presenting with neuromuscular disease before or at birth. Orphanet Journal of Rare Diseases. 2015;**10**(1). DOI: 10.1186/s13023-015-0364-0

[4] Bodkin C, Comer A, Felker M, Gutmann L, Jones K, Kincaid J, et al. Challenging neuromuscular disease cases. Seminars in Neurology. 2022;**42**(06):716-722. DOI: 10.1055/a-1985-0230

[5] Schöser B, Dusl M, Gallenmüller C, Guergueltcheva V, Schara U, Marina A, et al. Congenital myasthenic syndromes: Achievements and limitations of phenotype-guided gene-after-gene sequencing in diagnostic practice: A study of 680 patients. Human Mutation. 2012;**33**(10):1474-1484. DOI: 10.1002/humu.22130

[6] Scoto M, Finkel R, Mercuri E, Muntoni F. Genetic therapies for inherited neuromuscular disorders. The Lancet Child & Adolescent Health. 2018;**2**(8):600-609. DOI: 10.1016/s2352-4642(18)30140-8

[7] Hafeez K, Shaibani A. Diagnostic outcome of genetic testing for neuromuscular disorders in a tertiary center. Journal of Clinical Neuromuscular Disease. 2022;**24**(1):1-6. DOI: 10.1097/cnd.0000000000000389

[8] Barp A, Mosca L, SansoneV. Facilitations and hurdles of genetic testing in neuromuscular disorders. Diagnostics. 2021;**11**(4):701. DOI: 10.3390/diagnostics11040701

[9] Kiselev A, Vaz R, Knyazeva A, Sergushichev A, Dmitrieva R, Khudiakov A, et al. Truncating variant in myof gene is associated with limb-girdle type muscular dystrophy and cardiomyopathy. Frontiers in Genetics. 2019:10. DOI: 10.3389/fgene.2019.00608

[10] Ng K, Chin H, Chin A, Goh D. Using gene panels in the diagnosis of neuromuscular disorders: A mini-review. Frontiers in Neurology. 2022:13. DOI: 10.3389/fneur.2022.997551

[11] Winder T, Tan C, Klemm S, White H, Westbrook J, Wang J, et al. Clinical utility of multigene analysis in over 25,000 patients with neuromuscular disorders. Neurology Genetics. 2020;**6**(2). DOI: 10.1212/nxg.0000000000000412

[12] Laurent M. Crispr-based gene therapies: From preclinical to clinical treatments. Cells. 2024;**13**(10):800. DOI: 10.3390/cells13100800

[13] Ousterout D, Gersbach C. Genome Editing for Neuromuscular Diseases. 2016. pp. 51-79. DOI: 10.1007/978-1-4939-3509-3_4

[14] Hauschild L. Co-occurrence of myotonic dystrophy type 1 and limb-girdle muscular dystrophy

type 2b: A case report. Molecular Syndromology. 2023;**15**(1):58-62. DOI: 10.1159/000533219

[15] Garmendia J. Cns involvement in myotonic dystrophy type 1: Does sex play a role? Frontiers in Neurology. 2024:15. DOI: 10.3389/fneur.2024.1399898

[16] Torabi A. Unravelling the complexity of dysferlinopathy: A case report highlighting digenic inheritance of dysf and myh7 mutations. Biomedical Journal of Scientific & Technical Research. 2023;**53**(2) https://doi.org/10.26717/bjstr.2023.53.008388

[17] Chung B, Wong V, Ip P. Prevalence of neuromuscular diseases in Chinese children: A study in southern China. Journal of Child Neurology. 2003;**18**(3):217-219. DOI: 10.1177/08830738030180030201

[18] Sanmaneechai O. Pediatric neuromuscular diseases prevalence in siriraj hospital, Thailand's largest tertiary referral hospital. Siriraj Medical Journal. 2020;**72**(2):125-131 https://doi.org/10.33192/smj.2020.17

[19] Mahungu A, Monnakgotla N, Nel M, Heckmann J. A review of the genetic spectrum of hereditary spastic paraplegias, inherited neuropathies and spinal muscular atrophies in Africans. Orphanet Journal of Rare Diseases. 2022;**17**(1). DOI: 10.1186/s13023-022-02280-2

[20] Gouveia S, Vázquez-Mosquera M, Hermida-Ameijeiras Á, Sánchez-Pintos P, Castro M, León S, et al. Rapid molecular diagnosis of genetically inherited neuromuscular disorders using next-generation sequencing technologies. Journal of Clinical Medicine. 2022;**11**(10):2750. DOI: 10.3390/jcm11102750

[21] Cesar S. Neuromuscular diseases with hypertrophic cardiomyopathy. Global Cardiology Science and Practice. 2018;**2018**(3) https://doi.org/10.21542/gcsp.2018.27

[22] Chen D. Genetic therapies and respiratory outcomes in patients with neuromuscular disease. Current Opinion in Pediatrics. 2024. DOI: 10.1097/mop.0000000000001352

[23] Mackenzie F, Romero R, Williams D, Gillingwater T, Hilton H, Dick J, et al. Upregulation of pkd1l2 provokes a complex neuromuscular disease in the mouse. Human Molecular Genetics. 2009;**18**(19):3553-3566. DOI: 10.1093/hmg/ddp304

[24] Pogson D, Telfer J, Wimbush S. Prolonged vecuronium neuromuscular blockade associated with charcotmarie tooth neuropathy. British Journal of Anaesthesia. 2000;**85**(6):914-917. DOI: 10.1093/bja/85.6.914

[25] Thompson R, Schöser B, Beeson D, Engel A, Eymard B, Maxime E, et al. A nomenclature and classification for the congenital myasthenic syndromes: Preparing for fair data in the genomic era. Orphanet Journal of Rare Diseases. 2018;**13**(1). DOI: 10.1186/s13023-018-0955-7

[26] Shibata Y, Yabe I, Matsushima M, Hashimoto N, Yamada T, Sasaki H. Investigating the role of genetic counseling in neuromuscular disease considering life events. Journal of Human Genetics. 2019;**64**(6):551-559. DOI: 10.1038/s10038-019-0590-8

[27] Mignan T, Targett M, Lowrie M. Classification of myasthenia gravis and congenital myasthenic syndromes in dogs and cats. Journal of Veterinary Internal Medicine. 2020;**34**(5):1707-1717. DOI: 10.1111/jvim.15855

[28] Fecek C, Emmady PD. Facioscapulohumeral muscular dystrophy. [updated 2023 Jun 26]. In: StatPearls [Internet]. Treasure Island (FL): StatPearls Publishing; 2024. Available from: https://www.ncbi.nlm.nih.gov/books/NBK559028/

[29] Zhong H, Zhao C, Luo S. HLA in myasthenia gravis: From superficial correlation to underlying mechanism. Autoimmunity Reviews. 2019;**18**(9):102349. DOI: 10.1016/j.autrev.2019.102349

[30] Np H, Kurniawan A, Tjiang M. Worsening muscle weakness in myasthenia gravis patient suffering dengue infection. Journal of Tropical Diseases. 2014;**02**(03). DOI: 10.4172/2329-891x.1000140

[31] Park E, Shim Y, Ha J, Shin J, Lee S, Cho J. Diagnosis of duchenne muscular dystrophy in a presymptomatic infant using next-generation sequencing and chromosomal microarray analysis: A case report. Children. 2021;**8**(5):377. DOI: 10.3390/children8050377

[32] Galimberti V, Tironi R, Lerario A, Scali M, Bo R, Rodolico C, et al. Value of insoluble pabpn1 accumulation in the diagnosis of oculopharyngeal muscular dystrophy. European Journal of Neurology. 2019;**27**(4):709-715. DOI: 10.1111/ene.14131

[33] Kana V, Kellenberger C, Klein A. Muscle magnetic resonance imaging of the lower limbs: Valuable diagnostic tool in the investigation of childhood neuromuscular disorders. Neuropediatrics. 2014;**45**(05):278-288. DOI: 10.1055/s-0034-1381954

[34] Waldrop M, Pastore M, Schrader R, Sites E, Tsao C, Flanigan K. Diagnostic utility of whole exome sequencing in the neuromuscular clinic. Neuropediatrics. 2019;**50**(02):096-102. DOI: 10.1055/s-0039-1677734

[35] OlorónP. Congenital lmna-related muscular dystrophy in paediatrics: Cardiac management in monozygotic twins. International Journal of Molecular Sciences. 2024;**25**(11):5836. DOI: 10.3390/ijms25115836

[36] Schiffer D, Brignolio F, Chiò A, Giordana M, Meineri P, Rosso M, et al. A follow-up study of 60 cases of chronic spinal muscular atrophy. Neurological Sciences. 1988;**9**(1):47-51. DOI: 10.1007/bf02334407

[37] Meyer A. Exome sequencing in the pediatric neuromuscular clinic leads to more frequent diagnosis of both neuromuscular and neurodevelopmental conditions. Muscle & Nerve. 2023;**68**(6):833-840. DOI: 10.1002/mus.27976

[38] Nishioka S, Filho M, Marie S, Zatz M, Costa R. Distrofiamiotônica e cardiopatia: comportamento dos eventosarrítmicos e dos distúrbios da condução. ArquivosBrasileiros De Cardiologia. 2005;**84**(4):330-336. DOI: 10.1590/s0066-782x2005000400011

[39] Han H, Lee S, Choi Y, Rose M, Park H. Validation of the individualized neuromuscular quality of life questionnaire in Korean patients with genetic neuromuscular diseases. Journal of Clinical Neurology. 2022;**18**(5):514. DOI: 10.3988/jcn.2022.18.5.514

[40] Vivekanandam V, Jayaseelan D, Hanna M. Covid-19 infection and vaccination in patients with skeletal muscle channelopathies. Muscle & Nerve. 2022;**66**(5):617-620. DOI: 10.1002/mus.27704

[41] Christophers B, Lopez M, Gupta V, Baylies M. Pediatric nemaline myopathy: A systematic review

using individual patient data. 2022. DOI: 10.1101/2022.01.31.22270131

[42] Jaffry M. Neonatal fc receptor inhibitor therapeutics in neuromuscular disease. Journal of Clinical Neuromuscular Disease. 2023;**24**(4):188-198. DOI: 10.1097/cnd.0000000000000451

[43] Comley L, Nijssen J, Nylén J, Hedlund E. Cross-disease comparison of amyotrophic lateral sclerosis and spinal muscular atrophy reveals conservation of selective vulnerability but differential neuromuscular junction pathology. The Journal of Comparative Neurology. 2015;**524**(7):1424-1442. DOI: 10.1002/cne.23917

[44] Bello-Haas VD. Physical therapy for individuals with amyotrophic lateral sclerosis: Current insights. Degenerative Neurological and Neuromuscular Disease. 2018;**8**:45-54. DOI: 10.2147/DNND.S146949

[45] Majmudar S, Wu J, Paganoni S. Rehabilitation in amyotrophic lateral sclerosis: Why it matters. Muscle & Nerve. 2014;**50**(1):4-13. DOI: 10.1002/mus.24202

[46] Paganoni S, Karam C, Joyce N, Bedlack R, Carter GT. Comprehensive rehabilitative care across the spectrum of amyotrophic lateral sclerosis. NeuroRehabilitation. 2015;**37**(1):53-68. DOI: 10.3233/NRE-151240

[47] Pinto S, Quintarelli S, Silani V. New technologies and amyotrophic lateral sclerosis—Which step forward rushed by the COVID-19 pandemic? Journal of the Neurological Sciences. 2020;**418**:117081. DOI: 10.1016/j.jns.2020.117081

[48] Pugliese R, Sala R, Regondi S, Beltrami B, Lunetta C. Emerging technologies for management of patients with amyotrophic lateral sclerosis: From telehealth to assistive robotics and neural interfaces. Journal of Neurology. 2022;**269**(6):2910-2921. DOI: 10.1007/s00415-022-10971-w

[49] Riva N, Domi T, Pozzi L, et al. Update on recent advances in amyotrophic lateral sclerosis. Journal of Neurology. 2024;**271**(7):4693-4723. DOI: 10.1007/s00415-024-12435-9

[50] Ceyhan-Birsoy O, Talim B, Swanson L, Karakaya M, Graff M, Beggs A, et al. Whole exome sequencing reveals dysf, fktn, and ispd mutations in congenital muscular dystrophy without brain or eye involvement. Journal of Neuromuscular Diseases. 2015;**2**(1):87-92. DOI: 10.3233/jnd-140038

[51] Powis R, Karyka E, Boyd P, Come J, Jones R, Zheng Y, et al. Systemic restoration of uba1 ameliorates disease in spinal muscular atrophy. Jci. Insight. 2016;**1**(11). DOI: 10.1172/jci.insight.87908

[52] Santoso J, McCain M. Neuromuscular disease modeling on a chip. Disease Models & Mechanisms. 2020;**13**(7). DOI: 10.1242/dmm.044867

[53] Gorokhova S, Cerino M, Mathieu Y, Courrier S, Desvignes J, Salgado D, et al. Comparing targeted exome and whole exome approaches for genetic diagnosis of neuromuscular disorders. Applied & Translational Genomics. 2015;**7**:26-31. DOI: 10.1016/j.atg.2015.07.006

[54] Farmakidis C, Dimachkie M, Pasnoor M, Barohn R. Immunosuppressive and immunomodulatory therapies for neuromuscular diseases. Part I: Traditional agents. Muscle & Nerve. 2019;**61**(1):5-16. DOI: 10.1002/mus.26708

[55] Goyenvalle A, Griffith G, Babbs A, Andaloussi S, Ezzat K, Avril A, et al. Functional correction in mouse models of muscular dystrophy using

exon-skipping tricyclo-dna oligomers. Nature Medicine. 2015;**21**(3):270-275. DOI: 10.1038/nm.3765

[56] Birnkrant D, Carter J. Cardiopulmonary phenotypic variability and discordance in duchenne muscular dystrophy: Implications for new therapies. Pediatric Pulmonology. 2020;**56**(4):738-746. DOI: 10.1002/ppul.25111

[57] Maruyama R, Yokota T. Molecular diagnosis and novel therapies for neuromuscular diseases. Journal of Personalized Medicine. 2020;**10**(3):129. DOI: 10.3390/jpm10030129

[58] Duddy W, Duguez S. Understanding neuromuscular health and disease: Advances in genetics, omics, and molecular function. Journal of Personalized Medicine. 2021;**11**(5):438. DOI: 10.3390/jpm11050438

[59] Piñeros-Fernández M. Artificial intelligence applications in the diagnosis of neuromuscular diseases: A narrative review. Cureus. 2023. DOI: 10.7759/cureus.48458

[60] Abreu N, Waldrop M. Overview of gene therapy in spinal muscular atrophy and duchenne muscular dystrophy. Pediatric Pulmonology. 2020;**56**(4):710-720. DOI: 10.1002/ppul.25055

[61] Salwa, Pasha S, Fatima W, Srinivasamurthy S. Gene therapies for spinal muscular atrophy and duchenne muscular dystrophy: A pathbreaking moment in therapeutics. Journal of Pharmaceutical Research International. 2022:15-35. DOI: 10.9734/jpri/2022/v34i53b7229

[62] Aguti S, Malerba A, Zhou H. The progress of aav-mediated gene therapy in neuromuscular disorders. Expert Opinion on Biological Therapy. 2018;**18**(6):681-693. DOI: 10.1080/14712598.2018.1479739

[63] Maani N, Karolczak S, Dowling J. Genetic therapy for congenital myopathies. Current Opinion in Neurology. 2021;**34**(5):727-737. DOI: 10.1097/wco.0000000000000978

[64] Vila O, Sgm U, Sp M, Williams D, Kamm R, et al. Quantification of human neuromuscular function through optogenetics. Theranostics. 2019;**9**(5):1232-1246. DOI: 10.7150/thno.25735

[65] Falzarano M, Rossi R, Grilli A, Fang M, Osman H, Sabatelli P, et al. Urine-derived stem cells express 571 neuromuscular disorders causing genes, making them a potential in vitro model for rare genetic diseases. Frontiers in Physiology. 2021:12. DOI: 10.3389/fphys.2021.716471

[66] Raga S, Wilmshurst J, Smuts I, Meldau S, Bardien S, Schoonen M, et al. A case for genomic medicine in south African paediatric patients with neuromuscular disease. Frontiers in Pediatrics. 2022:10. DOI: 10.3389/fped.2022.1033299

[67] Mahoney A, Handberg C. New medicine for neuromuscular diseases: An evolving paradox for patient and family hopes and expectations. Nursing Inquiry. 2022;**30**(2). DOI: 10.1111/nin.12527

[68] Tasker R, Darras B. Neuromuscular disorders. Current Opinion in Pediatrics. 2013;**25**(6):674-675. DOI: 10.1097/mop.0b013e328365de49

[69] Atalaia A. Euro-nmd registry: Federated fair infrastructure, innovative technologies and concepts of a patient-centred registry for rare neuromuscular disorders. Orphanet Journal of Rare Diseases. 2024;**19**(1). DOI: 10.1186/s13023-024-03059-3

Chapter 2

Myasthenia Gravis: Pathophysiology, Diagnosis, and Management

Hassan Doumiati and Fatima Rawas

Abstract

Myasthenia gravis (MG) is the most common condition affecting the neuromuscular junction. It is always considered to be a great mimicker, and the diagnosis can be quite challenging. It occurs due to antibodies attacking receptors in the postsynaptic neuromuscular junction. A key symptom of MG is muscle fatigable weakness, often impacting the oculo-bulbar muscles. The disorder is categorized based on antibody status and clinical features. Diagnosis involves patient history, neurological examination, and a combination of laboratory and electrodiagnostic tests. The treatment of MG consists of symptomatic treatment such as acetylcholinesterase inhibitors, rapid therapies such as IV Ig or plasma exchange, and long-term therapies with immunosuppressant treatments. It is important to remember that certain drugs might induce de novo MG while others might exacerbate MG symptoms.

Keywords: myasthenia gravis, neuromuscular junction, acetylcholine receptors, thymectomy, plasma exchange, diagnosis, treatment, pathophysiology

1. Introduction

Myasthenia Gravis is considered a rare disease. At the same time, it is a great mimicker. In order to make the correct diagnosis, it should be on our differential diagnosis so that the workup for MG will be ordered. In this chapter, we will explore the pathophysiology of MG, discuss the clinical features, classification, and diagnostic methods, and review the latest management strategies.

2. Pathophysiology of MG

Myasthenia gravis (MG) occurs due to an antibody-mediated reversible receptor blocking on the neuromuscular junction, primarily targeting the nicotinic acetylcholine receptor (AChR). Other antibodies that may be involved include those against muscle-specific tyrosine kinase (MuSK) and lipoprotein-related protein 4 (LRP4) [1].

In a subset of MG patients, striational antibodies have also been detected, including those targeting titin, the ryanodine receptor, and the alpha subunit of the voltage-gated potassium channel [2].

IntechOpen

Triple seronegative MG is diagnosed when no autoantibodies are detected in the serum, but the diagnosis is confirmed through others [1].

The process of antibody-induced damage to the AChR is explained by two processes. Initially, the antibody binds to the receptor, which can directly obstruct acetylcholine (ACh) from binding. Secondly, a complement-mediated attack occurs, leading to the destruction of AChRs and postjunctional folds. Finally, antibody binding can cause an increased removal of AChRs from the postsynaptic membrane, known as modulation. This results in a smaller endplate potential despite a normal ACh release but decreased binding of ACh to its receptor [3].

Studies have demonstrated that antibodies binding to AChR lead to complement deposition at the NMJ. These antibodies, primarily from the IgG1 and IgG3 subclasses, are responsible for activating complement and subsequently causing NMJ destruction [4].

2.1 Pathophysiology of thymus pathology and MG

The thymus, a primary lymphoid organ, generates immunocompetent T cells. With age, the thymus undergoes atrophy, leading to a decline in its functions. It is essential for the development of a normal immune system [5].

Pathological alterations in the thymus are found in more than 80% of patients with MG and can be identified using computerized tomography (CT) or magnetic resonance imaging (MRI) [6].

More than 50% of MG patients exhibit thymic hyperplasia and about 10–15% present with either a benign low-grade thymoma of the thymic epithelium or an invasive thymoma. Slightly more than 50% of patients with thymoma will have or develop MG, often showing more severe clinical symptoms and higher AChR antibody titers than those without thymoma [6, 7].

Cases reported in the literature have shown a strong correlation between thymoma and early-onset MG, male gender, and the presence of striational antibodies [8, 9].

Other studies have indicated that thymic abnormalities, including thymoma or thymic hyperplasia, are more commonly found in generalized MG than in ocular MG. These abnormalities are less frequently seen in MuSK MG and seronegative, LRP4 MG [6, 10].

The thymus gland plays a crucial role in the mechanism of MG AChR autoantibodies production. The four-step sequence of intrathymic pathogenesis includes (1) myogenic induction of thymic stem cells, which leads to the synthesis and expression of AChR on thymic myoid cells; (2) release of AChR from myoid cells, followed by uptake of myoid AChR by thymic antigen-presenting cells and immunogenic presentation; (3) recognition of immunogenically presented AChR by specific autoreactive T lymphocytes differentiating within the thymus; (4) migration of the activated AChR-specific T lymphocytes to the peripheral immune system, interacting with AChR-specific B cells to produce pathogenic anti-AChR autoantibodies [11].

These findings support the idea that in MG patients with thymic hyperplasia, the onset of the generation of AChR antibodies begin within the thymus.

Thymoma, a rare tumor of thymic epithelial cells, is linked to autoimmunity, because of altered self-antigens expression by the neoplastic cells, including epitopes similar to AChR, titin, and ryanodine receptors. Unlike thymic hyperplasia, thymomas do not significantly produce autoantibodies. Nevertheless, autoreactive T lymphocytes may multiply, and activate B lymphocytes to produce autoantibodies after leaving the tumor. This is why around 100% of patients with thymomatous MG have detectable serum AChR antibodies [7].

3. Classification of MG

MG patients are classified based on different clinical features, which aid in discussions about prognosis and treatment options. Ocular MG is restricted to symptoms such as ptosis and diplopia, whereas generalized MG is diagnosed when a patient has weakness in bulbar, limb, axial, and respiratory muscles. Bulbar weakness, in particular, causes significant morbidity and is therefore considered a component of generalized MG [1] (**Table 1**).

The type of autoantibodies detected in the serum categorizes MG patients; these types are antibodies against AChR, MuSK, and LRP4 receptors. Patients with negative serum for autoantibodies are considered seronegative MG. Identifying the specific antibodies is crucial because different antibody profiles may lead to varying clinical courses and responses to treatment [1] (**Table 2**).

In patients with antibodies to AChR, myasthenic weakness typically impacts the extraocular, bulbar, or proximal limb muscles (**Table 2**).

Some studies of MG patients with MuSK antibodies report equal incidence among males and females, while others indicate a predominance of females [6].

Anti-MuSK MG patients typically experience a severe presentation of the disease in comparison to other types of MG. This is due to early weakness of bulbar, neck, and respiratory muscles, and a fast disease progression, with an elevated risk of myasthenic crises, and a lower likelihood of having a purely ocular MG presentation (**Table 2**) [1].

As mentioned earlier, seronegative MG can comprise up to 34% of MG patients, varying by study and the ethnic background of the cohort. Estimates of the prevalence of LPR4 autoantibodies among seronegative MG patients vary significantly, ranging from 3–50%. These variations could be due to differences in ethnic groups, study methodologies, or the limitations of small sample sizes. Seronegative MG, whether or not LPR4 autoantibodies are present, displays clinical features, progression, and treatment responses similar to those of AChR MG [6].

Lastly, MG patients are categorized based on the age at which the disease first appears. There is a notable clinical distinction between late-onset MG (usually defined as onset after age 50) and early-onset MG. Better overall outcomes are found in late-onset MG compared to those with earlier onset (**Table 3**) [1]. Patients with

	Myasthenia gravis classification based on clinical picture	
Classes	**Ocular**	**Generalized**
Involved muscles	Ocular muscles	Ocular, bulbar, axial limb, respiratory muscles

Table 1.
Classification of myasthenia gravis based on clinical picture and involved muscles.

	Myasthenia gravis classification based on serum autoantibodies against			
Classes	**AChR**	**MuSK**	**LRP4**	**Seronegative**
Involved muscles	Extra ocular, Bulbar, Proximal Limb muscles	Early bulbar, respiratory, Neck muscles	Similar to AChR	

Table 2.
Classification of myasthenia gravis based on serum autoantibodies and involved muscles.

	Myasthenia Gravis classification based on disease onset	
Outcome	Early-onset <50 y.o	Late-onset >50 y.o
	Worse outcome	Better outcome

Table 3.
Classification of myasthenia gravis based on disease onset and associated outcome.

early-onset MG have a higher incidence of thymic hyperplasia, and thymectomy has been shown to improve clinical outcomes and reduce the need for immunotherapy. In contrast, thymic hyperplasia is rare in late-onset MG, and the response to thymectomy is generally less favorable [2].

4. Clinical features of MG

MG patients suffer from fatigable, painless muscle weakness. As the disorder is restricted to the NMJ, it does not impact mental state, sensory, or autonomic functions [3].

MG typically develops subacutely and reaches its peak severity within 2 years. Due to the dynamic nature of the neuromuscular junction, myasthenic symptoms can fluctuate during the day [6].

The most common symptoms in MG patients are weakness of ocular muscles causing ptosis and diplopia due to extraocular muscle (EOM) weakness; these findings are encountered in over 50% of patients at the time of diagnosis [3].

Nonspecific visual blurring can occur before diplopia due to minimal ocular misalignment. The extraocular muscles most commonly affected are the levator palpebrae and the medial rectus muscles. Various patterns of ophthalmoparesis may appear [6].

Bulbar weakness is the second most common type of weakness after extraocular weakness. This can lead to difficulties with chewing, swallowing, and speaking. Patients might experience fatigue and weakness in the muscles used for mastication, making it hard to keep the jaw closed after chewing [3].

Bulbar muscle weakness affects an estimated 40% of MG patients at some stage of their illness. This condition may lead to hypophonia from vocal cord paresis or weakness of the expiratory muscles, and the voice might have a nasal tone due to palatal muscle weakness, which causes nasal air leakage. Patients may also experience dysarthria from weakness in the lips, tongue, or cheeks. Additional problems may include difficulty managing food due to tongue weakness and a weak cough [6].

Weakness in facial muscles is commonly observed and can lead to dysarthria and sialorrhea. It may also impact pulmonary function test results due to a compromised oral seal [6].

In most MG patients, weakness of the neck flexors is more common and more severe than weakness of the neck extensors. Head drop is relatively common and may even be the initial symptom [6].

Limb weakness affects 20–30% of individuals with the condition, primarily targeting proximal muscles. The weakness can be multifocal or diffuse and may predominantly involve the ocular and bulbar muscles [6].

Ventilatory insufficiency is an uncommon early symptom of myasthenia gravis but can occur in a significant number of patients with untreated or resistant disease [6].

DOI: http://dx.doi.org/10.5772/intechopen.1007603

A myasthenia gravis (MG) crisis is marked by the need for ventilatory support due to weakness of the respiratory muscles in MG patients. This occurs in 10–20% of individuals with generalized MG at least once during their lifetime, often within the first 2 years after diagnosis [12].

The main indicator of an impending MG crisis is growing weakness in the respiratory and bulbar muscles. Risk factors that contribute to the need for extended ventilation and longer stays in the intensive care unit include older age, late-onset MG, severe MG before the crisis, and the presence of multiple comorbidities [12].

Independent risk factors for myasthenic crises include the presence of a thymoma, MuSK antibodies, high disease severity at diagnosis, and the presence of striational antibodies [12, 13].

Acute ventilatory failure in myasthenia gravis patients can result from a combination of inadequate airway protection, insufficient secretion clearance due to weakness in the laryngeal and pharyngeal muscles, and hypoventilation caused by weakness in the diaphragm, intercostal muscles, and accessory muscles [12, 14].

Weakness in the diaphragm and other respiratory muscles is the main cause of hypoventilation and CO_2 retention. While this weakness can be chronic, it often becomes more pronounced during acute exacerbations, necessitating prompt and intensive hospital care [12].

Symptoms of hypoventilation due to respiratory muscle weakness are nonspecific and can include sleep disturbances, daytime sleepiness, and headaches. In myasthenia gravis patients, shortness of breath can arise from multiple causes and does not necessarily indicate muscle weakness [12].

5. Bedside examination of MG patient

When examining a suspected or confirmed MG patient, several distinctive features should be noted. Since ptosis is a prevalent symptom of MG, it is advisable to document the baseline position of the upper eyelid and lid relative to the pupil [6].

To detect or exacerbate extraocular muscle weakness, the patient is asked to hold an upward or lateral gaze for 1 minute while observing for any drifting of the eyelid or eye position. Cogan's lid twitch is another sign considered relatively specific, though not necessarily sensitive, for MG assessment. In this maneuver, the patient is first instructed to look downward and then quickly shift their gaze to the primary position. Normally, the eyelid moves in sync with the eyeball. A positive sign is indicated by the eyelid overshooting the eyeball position, leading to transient scleral exposure and upper lid oscillation [6].

Another technique is employed for patients with noticeable unilateral ptosis. In this method, the physician lifts the affected eyelid, which may either reveal or worsen ptosis in the opposite eyelid. This phenomenon can be explained by Hering's law of equal innervation, which states that manual elevation of one lid reduces the supranuclear stimulation of the levator subnucleus that controls both levator palpebrae muscles. Thus, elevating the more affected eyelid decreases the need for supranuclear stimulation of this nucleus, affecting both the contralateral and ipsilateral levator palpebrae muscles [6].

The icepack test is the final assessment for evaluating ptosis. Due to the known physiological enhancement of neuromuscular transmission through cooling, applying an ice pack to the eyelid for 1 minute or less can significantly improve existing ptosis [6].

The sensitivity of the ice pack test is 80–95% and the specificity of it is 79–97%. The sensitivity is as low as 25% when the patient has mild ptosis. However, this sensitivity increases to 70% by inducing muscle fatigue with prolonged upgaze before conducting the test [1].

In myasthenia gravis, patients are assessed for limb weakness, and the examination is repeated after exercises targeting the shoulder and pelvic girdle muscles, such as shoulder elevation and squatting, to screen for fatigable muscle weakness.

Data indicate that the Single Breath Count test and neck flexor strength testing are useful tools for evaluating respiratory function at the bedside in MG patients [15].

The Single Breath Count Test (SBCT) involved asking subjects to take a deep breath and count as far as possible at a rate of about two counts per second. An SBCT result greater than 25 indicates normal respiratory muscle function. Neck flexor strength was more closely linked to respiratory function, likely due to their role as accessory muscles in respiration [16].

As the disorder is restricted to the NMJ, it does not impact mental state, sensory, or autonomic functions [3].

6. Diagnosis of MG

Myasthenia is a clinical diagnosis confirmed by the presence of one or more of the following:

1. Presence of autoantibodies against AChR or MuSK

2. Response to edrophonium

3. Confirmatory result on repetitive nerve stimulation (RNS) or single-fiber electromyography (SFEMG) [6].

6.1 Antibodies testing

AChRs Autoantibodies are found in around 80% of patients with generalized MG. This test in generalized MG has a specificity of 90% [1].

False-positive results in AChR-binding antibody testing, often associated with low antibody titers, have been reported in other autoimmune conditions such as systemic lupus erythematosus, Hashimoto thyroiditis, and rheumatoid arthritis [1].

MuSK antibodies are usually tested when anti-AChR antibodies are not found [1]. If all antibodies are negative, LRP4 antibodies testing may be considered.

Eighty percent of MG patients test positive for anti-AChR antibodies. Seven to fifteen percent of MG patients test positive for MuSK antibodies. Double seropositivity for both AChR and MuSK antibodies is uncommon [2, 6]. Around 34% of MG patients are seronegative (including MG with LRP4 Antibodies) (**Figure 1**) [6].

In generalized MG, anti-AChR antibodies are found in 80% of the cases, and in ocular MG anti-AChR are found in more than 50% of the cases (**Figure 3**) [1, 2].

In up to 40% of generalized MG seronegative for anti-AChR, anti-MuSK antibodies are detected (**Figures 2** and **3**) [2].

The prevalence of anti-MuSK antibodies in isolated ocular myasthenia gravis is very low. Case reports indicate that among 38 patients with purely ocular seronegative MG tested for anti-MuSK antibodies, all results were negative (**Figure 2**) [17, 18].

The concentration of anti-MuSK antibodies has a significant correlation with disease severity, making serum anti-MuSK IgG titers valuable biological markers for the disease. In contrast, AChR antibody titers do not generally correlate with disease severity, though there is some evidence suggesting a correlation when considering the IgG1 subclass. Tracking antibody titers can be highly useful for monitoring disease progression and response to treatment [19, 20].

6.2 Electrodiagnostic testing

For patients suspected of having MG who have negative antibody tests or who may have false-positive antibody results, electrodiagnostic testing is valuable. Evaluating MG typically includes routine nerve conduction studies and EMG, exercise testing, repetitive nerve stimulation (RNS), and single-fiber EMG (SF-EMG) [1, 3].

6.2.1 Nerve conduction studies

Motor and sensory conduction studies should be carried out for both upper and lower extremities.

Normal CMAP amplitudes are expected in MG, whereas in LEMS, they are typically diffusely low [3].

Routine nerve conduction studies must confirm that the nerve remains intact before it undergoes repetitive nerve stimulation testing (RNS) [3].

6.2.2 Repetitive nerve stimulation

RNS are abnormal in over 50–70% of generalized MG patients and are commonly normal in localized ocular MG [3].

A decremental response on repetitive nerve stimulation reflects clinical muscle fatigue and weakness. A CMAP decrement of 10% or more during slow (3 Hz) RNS is typically observed in MG [3].

Both distal and proximal nerves should be examined. Facial RNS is particularly crucial in suspected anti-MuSK antibody-associated MG due to the severe bulbar and facial involvement seen in these patients [3].

In generalized MG slow RNS testing (at 2–3 Hz) has a 40–50% sensitivity and 95–100% specificity [1].

6.2.3 Exercise testing

If there is no decrement or a decrement of less than 10% on baseline RNS studies, the patient undergoes 1 minute of exercise, followed by RNS at 1-minute intervals for 3–4 minutes, to check for a post-exercise fatigue-induced decrease in CMAP [3].

6.2.4 Electromyography

Generally, needle EMG findings in neuromuscular junction disorders appear normal. EMG is conducted for two primary reasons: First, to rule out severe denervating disorders and myotonic disorders that could also show a decreased CMAP response on repetitive nerve stimulation. The needle EMG may identify unstable motor unit action potentials (MUAPs) and/or small, short-duration MUAPs that resemble myopathic MUAPs [3].

6.2.5 Single-fiber electromyography

In generalized MG, single-fiber EMG sensitivity is around 75–90% and specificity ranges from 60–90%. This test evaluates the non-synchronous firing of muscle fibers within the same motor unit, resulting in the electrical observation of increased jitter [1].

False-positive results can occur in neuropathies, myopathies, and motor neuron disease. Therefore, it is essential to correlate single-fiber EMG findings with the clinical presentation [1].

The primary advantage of single-fiber EMG (SF-EMG) over repetitive nerve stimulation (RNS) is that SF-EMG can reveal abnormalities, such as increased jitter, even in patients who do not exhibit overt clinical weakness [3].

7. Treatment of MG

7.1 Treatment goals

The treatment of patients with MG aims at abolishing or decreasing the symptoms of the disease. An important goal is to keep the patients in their full functional capacity avoiding fluctuations in their symptoms or exacerbations. A further important goal is to improve compliance to medications by taking into consideration the short and long-term side effects of the medications used and to adjust the dosages accordingly.

7.2 Overview of therapies

7.2.1 Symptomatic treatment

Oral acetylcholinesterase (AChE) inhibitors increase the acetylcholine amount at the neuromuscular junction. They are recommended as first-line therapy for MG. Pyridostigmine is the most commonly used. It is generally considered as safe. It can be used as a single long-term treatment in patients with generalized stable mild disease and as an add-on therapy in patients with severe disease whose conditions require adding immunotherapy [21].

Pyridostigmine begins to take effect about 15–30 minutes after ingestion, with its peak action occurring approximately 2 hours after administration. The effects typically last for three to 4 hours, and occasionally longer.

Choosing among the treatments depends on the severity and the pace of the disease and it is tailored according to each case.

Patients whose disease is well controlled on pyridostigmine alone are followed clinically. While some patients manage well with pyridostigmine alone for long-term treatment, the majority of those with generalized MG eventually need additional therapy at some stage of their illness or for the rest of their lives [22].

7.2.2 Rapid therapies

These therapies start to show effects within a few days, but their benefits typically last only a few weeks. They include plasma exchange and intravenous immune globulin.

Plasma exchange, or plasmapheresis, effectively removes acetylcholine receptor antibodies from the bloodstream and is commonly used to manage myasthenic crises. The improvement typically lasts for 3–4 weeks. It is important to note that antibody levels may rebound within weeks if immunosuppressants are not used concurrently. The treatment generally involves five exchanges, each removing 3 to 5 liters of plasma, performed every other day over the course of 1–2 weeks [22].

Intravenous immune globulin (IVIG) is employed similarly to plasma exchange for treating myasthenia exacerbations. IVIG is made up of pooled immunoglobulins from numerous donors. Its exact mechanism of action in myasthenia is not well understood. The typical dosage is 2 g/kg, administered over a period of 2–5 days.

7.2.3 Chronic long-term immunotherapies

It is indicated to start immunotherapy for patients who are still symptomatic despite being on pyridostigmine, or whom relief after taking pyridostigmine is temporary. Typically, management starts with the addition of glucocorticoids. However, many patients with generalized MG will also need to incorporate a nonsteroidal immunotherapeutic agent, such as azathioprine or mycophenolate, to mitigate the long-term side effects of glucocorticoids [22].

7.2.3.1 Glucocorticoids

Glucocorticoids are the preferred choice for initial immunosuppressive therapy due to their rapid onset of effect. For patients at higher risk of glucocorticoid-related complications, we aim to shorten the duration of the initial prednisone treatment or avoid glucocorticoids altogether. This may involve early initiation of a nonsteroidal immunosuppressive therapy, such as azathioprine or mycophenolate, and using bridge therapies like intravenous immune globulin (IVIG) or plasmapheresis. The approach should be tailored based on the disease severity and specific comorbid risk factors [22].

Prednisone is typically initiated at a dose of 20 mg daily, with increments of 5 mg every 3–5 days until reaching 1 mg/kg per day (not more than 80 mg daily). This process usually takes 4–8 weeks, to be able to evaluate the effectiveness of the steroids. After about a month at this dosage, tapering can commence [22].

The aim should be to reduce the prednisone dose to 7.5 mg/day within 1 year.

Patients on 7.5 mg/day of prednisone with minimal disease symptoms tend to experience a better quality of life and report fewer side effects compared to those on higher doses [1].

When high-dose glucocorticoids are initiated, up to 50% of patients may experience a temporary worsening of their condition, which can be severe [22].

For more severely affected patients in whom corticosteroids are contraindicated, treatments such as IVIg, plasma exchange, or eculizumab may be considered as a bridging therapy until non-corticosteroid oral agents become effective [1].

Immunotherapies are frequently used in conjunction with glucocorticoids due to inadequate response, difficulties in tapering glucocorticoids without symptom recurrence, or the development of toxicities from long-term steroid use [22].

7.2.3.2 Glucocorticoid-sparing therapy

The most commonly used glucocorticoid-sparing therapies are azathioprine and mycophenolate mofetil. These oral non-corticosteroid immunosuppressive agents are not typically effective until 1–14 months after initiating therapy [22].

7.2.3.3 Rituximab

Rituximab which is administered via intravenous infusion, is a human/murine chimeric monoclonal antibody against the CD20 protein. There is enough evidence about benefit of rituximab therapy in MG patients who are MuSK-positive. Rituximab is a therapeutic option even ahead of conventional immunosuppressants. The ideal dose and dosing schedule for rituximab remain debated. A typical starting regimen is 375 mg/m^2 weekly for 4 weeks, while another approach involves administering a fixed dose of 1000 mg, repeating it in 2 weeks for a total of 2000 mg, followed by 1 g every 6 months [23].

7.2.3.4 Eculizumab

Eculizumab, a monoclonal antibody targeting complement C5, is the first complement inhibitor approved by the FDA for the treatment of refractory anti-AChR-positive myasthenia gravis. Clinical improvements typically begin within 2 weeks after the initial infusion, reach their peak at around 3 months for most patients, and remain stable for at least 3 years [1].

In AChR antibody-positive MG, which causes postsynaptic damage through complement cascade activation, eculizumab functions by blocking the formation of C5b. This inhibition helps prevent the formation of the membrane attack complex. Additionally, eculizumab blocks the production of C5a, a powerful pro-inflammatory and anaphylactic mediator [24].

Eculizumab is infused intravenously over 35 minutes in adults, starting with 900 mg weekly for the first four doses. After that, the dosage is increased to 1200 mg 1 week later and then continued at 1200 mg every 2 weeks [24].

7.2.3.5 Selection of therapy

For AChR-positive and seronegative MG, azathioprine and mycophenolate mofetil are the most commonly used therapies to reduce reliance on glucocorticoids.

MuSK-positive MG: International expert consensus guidelines highlight key differences between MuSK-positive myasthenia gravis (MG), AChR antibody-positive, and seronegative MG treatment regimens. Most patients with MuSK-positive MG have a limited response to anticholinesterase medications. Although many do respond to glucocorticoids, they often remain reliant on steroids, even with the addition of other immunosuppressants like azathioprine or mycophenolate mofetil. Rituximab has become a preferred early treatment, particularly if glucocorticoids are insufficient. Since IVIG is less effective than plasma exchange in this group, the three most effective treatments for MuSK-positive MG are corticosteroids, rituximab, and plasma exchange [22].

IVIG and plasma exchange can be used as a short-term therapy for Moderate to severe MG, aiming to provide rapid improvement and act as a bridge to prednisone or other immunosuppressants with a slower onset of action. It can also serve as maintenance therapy for patients who have poor responses to or cannot tolerate multiple immunosuppressants, as well as in preoperative settings to optimize patient strength and in cases of impending or active MG crisis [1].

7.2.4 Thymectomy

In the treatment of myasthenia gravis, thymectomy has its role in parallel with symptomatic therapy and immune therapy.

Patients with thymoma: 10–15% of patients with MG have a thymoma, and it is an indication to do thymectomy when it is feasible. When it is not feasible, chemotherapy and radiation are alternatives.

The role of thymectomy in patients without AChR antibodies or in older individuals is more debated, and treatment decisions are tailored to each individual.

Thymectomy is not recommended for patients with anti-MuSK or ocular MG. However, the landmark MGTX trial demonstrated significant and long-lasting benefits of thymectomy in non-thymomatous patients with anti-AChR-positive generalized MG who are under 50 years of age [1].

7.2.5 Rehabilitation therapy

MG significantly affects the physical and social well-being of patients, leading to a reduced quality of life. Rehabilitation, designed to help individuals with disabilities attain optimal quality of life and maintain functional independence, plays a crucial role in the multidisciplinary care of MG patients, being both safe and effective.

A well-structured rehabilitation program can help reduce secondary medical conditions and manage potential MG complications respiratory failure [25].

Research shows that rehabilitative methods, including physical and respiratory muscle training, help alleviate fatigue and improve the quality of life for MG patients [25].

Another observational study shows that a structured program of physical and respiratory rehabilitation therapy can be successfully applied to myasthenic patients for both preoperative preparation and postoperative recovery following thymectomy surgery. Rehabilitation programs improved key parameters affected by MG, such as MG quantitative score (13-item direct physician assessment scoring system that quantifies disease severity based on impairments of body functions and structures), fatigue score, physical function, walking endurance, and lung capacity. These improvements were notably greater than those in a matched control group without rehabilitation. Furthermore, the rehabilitation group experienced shorter postoperative recovery times, lower rates of major complications, fewer intensive care unit (ICU) admissions, and shorter hospital stays [26].

The greatest benefits of physical training have been seen in patients with mild to moderate MG, particularly when done at a controlled intensity to prevent muscle fatigue. It has been especially effective in preventing muscle atrophy due to disuse and in preserving muscle strength [25].

Respiratory training was found highly effective in strengthening respiratory muscles, improving endurance, and reducing dyspnea. Its effectiveness is attributed to long-term endurance training, which lowers respiratory rates, reduces the effort of breathing, and ultimately enhances physical fitness [25].

7.3 Response assessment

It is important to document baseline neurological function and examination, which should be monitored over time as therapies are introduced or adjusted. The effectiveness of treatments is assessed by observing improvements in clinical symptoms and neurological deficits during examinations [22].

Because AChR antibody titers do not correlate with disease severity, acetylcholine receptors (AChRs) are not recommended as markers for treatment response in myasthenia gravis (MG). However, as noted earlier, anti-MuSK antibody titers are considered reliable markers for treatment response due to their correlation with disease severity [22].

7.4 Acute exacerbations

Myasthenic symptoms may temporarily worsen over time. Common triggers for this include acute infections, surgery, pregnancy, childbirth, certain medications, tapering of immunotherapeutic drugs, or spontaneously as part of the disease's natural progression [22].

Acute exacerbations can be divided into two parts depending on the severity of symptoms: Myasthenic crisis and less severe exacerbations.

Myasthenic crisis: As previously noted, patients in a myasthenic crisis often experience widespread weakness with respiratory insufficiency that is disproportionate to their limb or bulbar weakness. Once respiratory support is provided, acute management of the crisis involves plasma exchange or IVIG. Pyridostigmine is typically withheld to minimize oropharyngeal secretions. If symptomatic treatment is insufficient, steroid therapy, such as prednisone, may be started. Steroid-sparing agents should be considered to mitigate potential adverse effects [24].

Less severe exacerbations: Patients with MG often experience a worsening of symptoms that is not severe enough to qualify as a myasthenic crisis.

In both types of exacerbations, the initial step is to address any external factors contributing to the exacerbation, such as treating a concurrent infection or discontinuing a medication that may worsen myasthenia [22].

The treatment approach should be tailored to the patient's specific symptoms, considering the rate of neurological decline, the presence of dysphagia, dyspnea, and other significant functional limitations. Treatment settings can range from outpatient care to inpatient or even intensive care unit (ICU) admission, depending on symptom severity and progression [22].

For mild exacerbations (e.g., mild ptosis, diplopia, facial or limb weakness, or mild dysarthria), treatment may involve increasing the dose of pyridostigmine, initiating or adjusting glucocorticoid therapy, or closely monitoring the patient while addressing any secondary causes of the exacerbation.

In cases of worsening dysphagia or dyspnea with the potential for a myasthenic crisis, ICU admission may be necessary. Treatment in this scenario is managed similarly to a myasthenic crisis [22].

7.5 Avoiding medications that could worsen myasthenia

A number of medications precipitate autoimmunity and therefore may induce de novo MG such as immune checkpoint inhibitors, penicillamine, tyrosine kinase inhibitors, and interferons.

Many more drugs such as certain antibiotics (macrolides, fluoroquinolones, aminoglycosides, etc.), antiarrhythmics, anesthetics, and neuromuscular blockers adversely affect the neuromuscular junction transmission and have been implicated in worsening of MG symptomatology, including precipitation of MG crisis, or unmasking of a previously undiagnosed MG [27].

7.6 Immunizations

Patients with generalized MG who develop respiratory infections face a higher risk of exacerbations and respiratory failure [28]. Current guidelines advise annual seasonal influenza vaccination (preferably with the inactivated vaccine) for individuals on immunosuppressive therapy, as well as for those with neurological conditions that impair secretion management, including neuromuscular disorders like generalized MG or ocular MG within 3 years of onset, due to the risk of progression to generalized MG [22].

8. Conclusion

Myasthenia Gravis (MG) is a neuromuscular disorder characterized by muscle weakness, which is typically caused by antibodies that attack receptors in the postsynaptic neuromuscular junction. Myasthenia Gravis is a great mimicker. It should be on the list of the differential diagnosis of certain symptoms in certain conditions such as diplopia, dysphagia, dysarthria, and ptosis in order to do the work up.

The classification of MG is based on clinical features and the presence of specific autoantibodies such as anti-AChR, anti-MuSK, and LRP4. The diagnostic process involves a combination of patient history, neurological examination, and various laboratory and electrodiagnostic tests to confirm the condition and determine its specific type.

Treatment for MG varies based on the severity and antibody profile.

Acetylcholinesterase inhibitors, corticosteroids, and immunosuppressants are commonly used to manage symptoms and slow disease progression. Plasma exchange and intravenous immunoglobulin (IVIG) are often considered for rapid relief in cases of crisis or severe exacerbation. Rituximab and eculizumab have shown particular effectiveness in patients with specific antibody profiles, such as anti-MuSK or refractory anti-AChR-positive MG, offering new avenues for treatment.

Long-term management of MG focuses on minimizing symptoms, improving quality of life, and reducing medication side effects, with thymectomy recommended for certain subtypes, especially younger patients with anti-AChR-positive generalized MG. A personalized treatment approach and regular monitoring are essential to adapt therapies to individual needs. Additionally, rehabilitation, particularly structured physical and respiratory programs, plays a crucial role in enhancing quality of life, preventing muscle atrophy, improving respiratory function, and reducing complications, especially in surgical recovery.

Acknowledgements

We extend our heartfelt gratitude to our families for their unwavering support. A special thanks goes to our teacher, Professor Raja Sawaya, for reviewing the chapter and providing valuable feedback.

Conflict of interest

The authors declare no conflict of interest.

Nomenclature

AChR	acetylcholine receptor
MuSK	muscle-specific kinase
LRP4	low-density lipoprotein receptor-related protein 4
IVIG	intravenous immunoglobulin
MG	myasthenia gravis

NMJ	neuromuscular junction
CMAP	compound muscle action potential
SFEMG	single-fiber electromyography

A. Appendix

Figure 1 showing the percentages of seropositive and seronegative myasthenia gravis (MG) cases, including anti-AChR (80%), Anti-MuSK (11%), and seronegative (including LRP4) cases (34%).

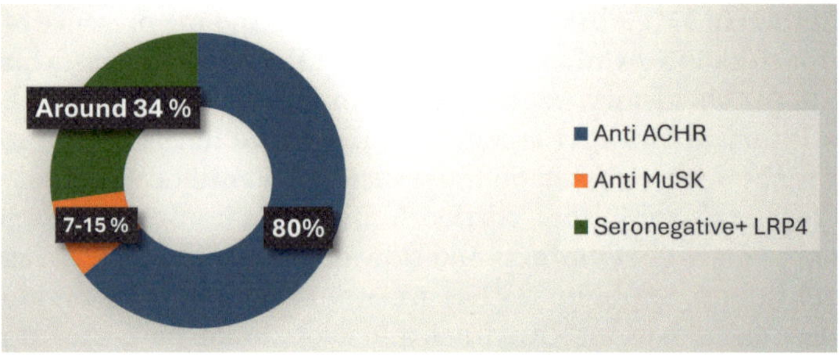

Figure 1.
MG seropositive and seronegative percentages.

B. Appendix

Figure 2 showing the distribution of seropositive antibodies in ocular MG cases.

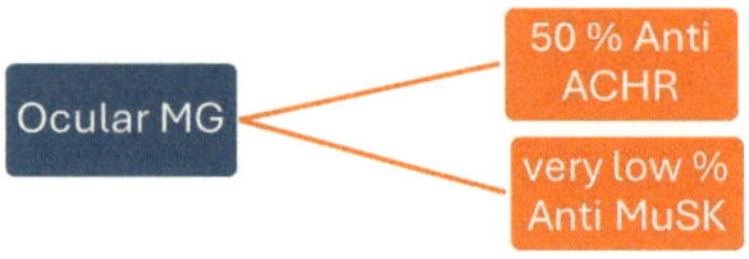

Figure 2.
Seropositive antibodies in Ocular MG.

C. Appendix

Figure 3 illustrating the distribution of seropositive antibodies in generalized MG cases.

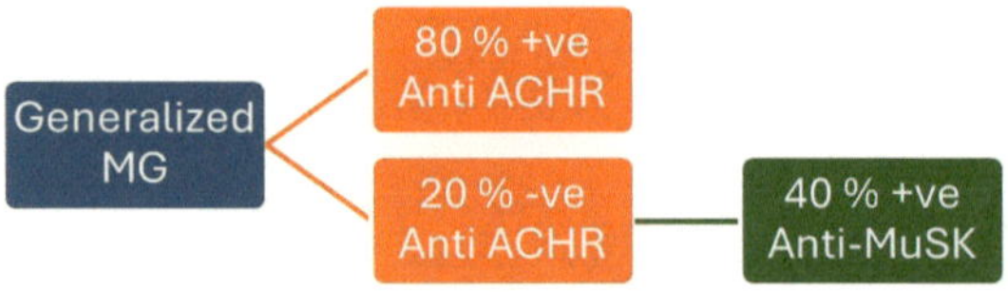
Generalized MG
80 % +ve Anti ACHR
20 % -ve Anti ACHR
40 % +ve Anti-MuSK

Figure 3.
Seropositive antibodies in Generalized MG.

Author details

Hassan Doumiati* and Fatima Rawas
American University of Beirut Medical Center, Lebanon

*Address all correspondence to: hd32@aub.edu.lb

References

[1] Hehir MK 2nd, LI Y. Diagnosis and Management of Myasthenia Gravis. Continuum (Minneapolis Minnesota). 2022;**28**(6):1615-1642

[2] Dresser L, Wlodarski R, Rezania K, Soliven B. Myasthenia gravis: Epidemiology, pathophysiology and clinical manifestations. Journal of Clinical Medicine. 2021;**10**(11):2235. DOI: 10.3390/jcm10112235

[3] Electromyography and Neuromuscular Disorders. Clinical-Electrophysiologic Ultrasound Correlations. 4th ed. Preston: Shapiro; 2021

[4] San PP, Jacob S. Role of complement in myasthenia gravis. Frontiers in Neurology. 2023;**14**:1277596. DOI: 10.3389/fneur.2023.1277596

[5] Rezzani R, Nardo L, Favero G, Peroni M, Rodella LF. Thymus and aging: Morphological, radiological, and functional overview. Age (Dordrecht, Netherlands). 2014;**36**(1):313-351

[6] Amato AA, Russell JA. Neuromuscular disorders. 2nd ed.; 2016

[7] Meriggioli MN, Sanders DB. Muscle autoantibodies in myasthenia gravis: Beyond diagnosis? Expert Review of Clinical Immunology. 2012;**8**(5):427-438

[8] Bernard C, Frih H, Pasquet F, Kerever S, Jamilloux Y, Tronc F, et al. Thymoma associated with autoimmune diseases: 85 cases and literature review. Autoimmunity Reviews. 2016;**15**(1):82-92. DOI: 10.1016/j.autrev.2015.09.005

[9] Mao ZF, Mo XA, Qin C, Lai YR, Hackett ML. Incidence of thymoma in myasthenia gravis: A systematic review. Journal of Clinical Neurology. 2012;**8**(3):161-169. DOI: 10.3988/jcn.2012.8.3.161

[10] Hsu SY, Tsai RK, Wang HZ, Su MY. A comparative study of ocular and generalized myasthenia gravis. The Kaohsiung Journal of Medical Sciences. 2002;**18**(2):62-69

[11] Melms A, Schalke BC, Kirchner T, Müller-Hermelink HK, Albert E, Wekerle H. Thymus in myasthenia gravis. Isolation of T-lymphocyte lines specific for the nicotinic acetylcholine receptor from thymuses of myasthenic patients. The Journal of Clinical Investigation. 1988;**81**(3):902-908

[12] Gilhus NE. Myasthenia gravis, respiratory function, and respiratory tract disease. Journal of Neurology. 2023;**270**(7):3329-3340

[13] Nelke C, Stascheit F, Eckert C, Pawlitzki M, Schroeter CB, Huntemann N, et al. Independent risk factors for myasthenic crisis and disease exacerbation in a retrospective cohort of myasthenia gravis patients. Journal of Neuroinflammation. 2022;**19**(1):89. DOI: 10.1186/s12974-022-02448-4

[14] Borel CO, Tilford C, Nichols DG, Hanley DF, Traystman RJ. Diaphragmatic performance during recovery from acute ventilatory failure in Guillain-Barré syndrome and myasthenia gravis. Chest. 1991;**99**(2):444-451

[15] Elsheikh B, Arnold WD, Gharibshahi S, Reynolds J, Freimer M, Kissel JT. Correlation of single-breath count test and neck flexor muscle strength with spirometry in myasthenia gravis. Muscle & Nerve. 2016;**53**(1):134-136. DOI: 10.1002/mus.24929

[16] Elsheikh B, Arnold WD, Gharibshahi S, Reynolds J, Freimer M, Kissel JT. Correlation of single-breath count test and neck flexor muscle strength with spirometry in myasthenia gravis. Muscle & Nerve. 2016;**53**(1):134-136. DOI: 10.1002/mus.24929

[17] Bennett DL, Mills KR, Riordan-Eva P, Barnes PR, Rose MR. Anti-MuSK antibodies in a case of ocular myasthenia gravis. Journal of Neurology, Neurosurgery, and Psychiatry. 2006;**77**(4):564-565. DOI: 10.1136/jnnp.2005.075812

[18] Caress JB, Hunt CH, Batish SD. Anti-MuSK myasthenia gravis presenting with purely ocular findings. Archives of Neurology. 2005;**62**(6):1002-1003. DOI: 10.1001/archneur.62.6.1002

[19] Bartoccioni E, Scuderi F, Minicuci GM, Marino M, Ciaraffa F, Evoli A. Anti-MuSK antibodies: Correlation with myasthenia gravis severity. Neurology. 2006;**67**(3):505-507. DOI: 10.1212/01.wnl.0000228225.23349.5d

[20] Lazaridis K, Tzartos SJ. Autoantibody specificities in myasthenia gravis; implications for improved diagnostics and therapeutics. Frontiers in Immunology. 2020;**11**:212. DOI: 10.3389/fimmu.2020.00212

[21] Maggi L, Mantegazza R. Treatment of myasthenia gravis: Focus on pyridostigmine. Clinical Drug Investigation. 2011;**31**(10):691-701. DOI: 10.2165/11593300-000000000-00000

[22] Shwan J, Bird MD. In: Goddeau RP, editor. Overview of the treatment of myasthenia gravis. Uptodate; 2024. Available from: www.uptodate.com/contents/overview-of-the-treatment-of-myasthenia-gravis

[23] Vesperinas-Castro A, Cortés-Vicente E. Rituximab treatment in myasthenia gravis. Frontiers in Neurology. 2023;**14**:1275533. DOI: 10.3389/fneur.2023.1275533

[24] Zhou A, Ho S, Vickers A. Eculizumab in myasthenia gravis: A review. Saudi Journal of Ophthalmology. 2024;**38**(1):34-40. DOI: 10.4103/sjopt.sjopt_74_23

[25] Corrado B, Giardulli B, Costa M. Evidence-based practice in rehabilitation of myasthenia gravis. A systematic review of the literature. Journal of Functional Morphology and Kinesiology. 2020;**5**(4):71. DOI: 10.3390/jfmk5040071

[26] Ambrogi V, Mineo TC. Benefits of comprehensive rehabilitation therapy in thymectomy for myasthenia gravis: A propensity score matching analysis. American Journal of Physical Medicine and Rehabilitation. 2017;**96**(2):77-83. DOI: 10.1097/PHM.0000000000000538

[27] Sheikh S, Alvi U, Soliven B, Rezania K. Drugs that induce or cause deterioration of myasthenia gravis: An update. Journal of Clinical Medicine. 2021;**10**(7):1537. DOI: 10.3390/jcm10071537

[28] Thomas CE, Mayer SA, Gungor Y, Swarup R, Webster EA, Chang I, et al. Myasthenic crisis: Clinical features, mortality, complications, and risk factors for prolonged intubation. Neurology. 1997;**48**(5):1253-1260. DOI: 10.1212/wnl.48.5.1253

Chapter 3

Expiratory Muscle Training in Motor Neuron Diseases: Impact on the Upper Airways

Alessandra Carneiro Dorça and Letícia de Araújo Morais

Abstract

Amyotrophic lateral sclerosis (ALS) is a progressive and idiopathic neurodegenerative disease with no known cure, influenced by a variety of factors. The survival of individuals with ALS is closely tied to the effective management of symptoms, particularly the preservation of respiratory and motor functions. This chapter focuses on the importance of clinical protocols designed to delay respiratory deterioration, emphasizing the role of noninvasive ventilation (NIV) and upper airway expiratory techniques in extending survival and enhancing the quality of life. Multidisciplinary approaches in ALS care aim to postpone the need for tracheostomy, with a central focus on NIV to optimize lung function and improve patient outcomes. The use of ventilators with mouthpiece interfaces contributes not only to respiratory safety but also to the preservation of voice quality. Additionally, expiratory muscle training enhances the strength of muscles involved in breathing, leading to significant improvements in respiratory function.

Keywords: amyotrophic lateral sclerosis, muscle training, noninvasive ventilation, motor neuron diseases, respiratory exercises

1. Introduction

Motor neuron diseases (MNDs), including amyotrophic lateral sclerosis (ALS), manifest in various ways. Moreover, respiratory changes play a crucial role in disease progression and patient survival [1]. Respiratory infection, secondary to impaired respiratory defenses, chest wall restriction, weak cough, and recurrent respiratory tract infections, is the leading cause of morbidity and mortality in this population.

ALS can be subdivided into bulbar onset and limb onset based on the somatic region involved [2]. Respiratory complications are particularly prevalent and fatal in patients with bulbar-onset alS, accounting for more than 85% of deaths. In contrast, limb-onset alS is associated with longer survival, although respiratory dysfunction still occurs as the disease progresses [3].

Restrictive ventilatory impairment is a common feature in most MNDs. As the disease progresses and lung volumes decrease, individuals lose the ability to inhale and cough effectively, which can lead to hypercapnia, respiratory failure, and the need for home mechanical ventilation. Eventually, most individuals die due to these complications. The reduction in vital capacity (VC) is an indicator of respiratory muscle weakness, both inspiratory and expiratory, but the loss of lung volume tends to be greater than expected based solely on muscle weakness [4].

Multidisciplinary interventions for ALS patients aim to delay the need for tracheostomy, focusing on noninvasive ventilation (NIV), which improves survival and preserves lung capacity. Using ventilators with a mouthpiece attachment contributes to respiratory safety and enhances voice quality. Furthermore, expiratory muscle training targets the strengthening of the muscles involved in expiration, leading to improvements in respiratory variables [5, 6].

2. Functional respiratory changes in different phenotypes of MND

The ALS spectrum encompasses various clinical phenotypes, with variations in the degrees of involvement of upper motor neurons (UMNs) and lower motor neurons (LMNs), as well as extramotor manifestations, primarily frontotemporal. In the different phenotypes, respiratory manifestations can vary. In the case of limb-onset alS (appendicular), weakness typically begins in the distal muscles and progresses to the muscles responsible for pulmonary mechanics, resulting in alveolar hypoventilation and respiratory failure [7]. In contrast, bulbar-onset alS involves early engagement of the respiratory muscles, especially the diaphragm, leading to a rapid decrease in lung volumes, such as tidal volume (TV) and VC, culminating in hypercapnia and respiratory failure (**Figure 1**) [8].

The weakness resulting from the degeneration of LMNs underlying ALS leads to a reduction in the ability to generate intrathoracic pressure, decreased chest expansion during inhalation, and diminished elastic recoil forces during exhalation. The involvement of UMNs in ALS causes rigidity of the chest wall, increasing resistance and limiting the range of motion, which functionally elevates the mechanical forces required to maintain adequate ventilation. In addition, the reduction in speed, range of motion, and weakness of the respiratory, laryngeal, and bulbar systems further affects the ability to clear the airways in individuals with ALS. Clinically, this manifests as difficulties in managing secretions, airway defense, and the effective expulsion of tracheal contents [8].

Respiratory manifestations, regardless of the phenotype, include exacerbated dyspnea during exertion and at rest, orthopnea, sleep-related breathing disorders,

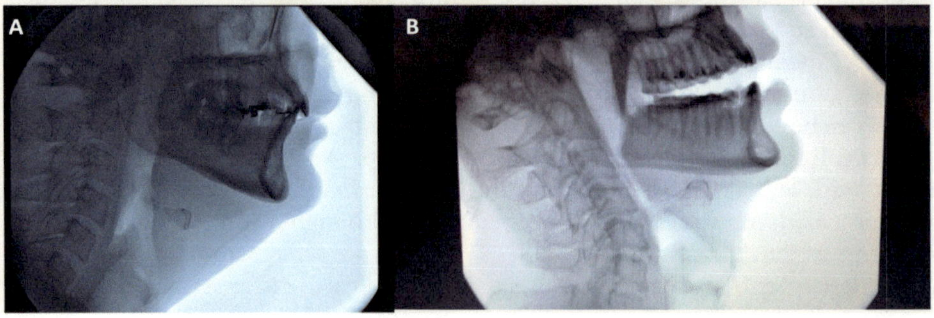

Figure 1.
Videofluoroscopy at rest of individuals with ALS. A: Individual with limb-onset (appendicular) ALS, 89% forced vital capacity; B: Individual with bulbar-onset alS, 12% forced vital capacity. Source: personal collection.

and weakness of the expiratory muscles, which compromises the ability to cough and clear secretions. Using accessory muscles for breathing and paradoxical breathing are typical clinical signs observed during disease progression [9].

3. An overview of respiratory changes and their consequences

3.1 Functional respiratory changes in ALS

In ALS, functional respiratory changes are one of the most critical manifestations of the disease, directly impacting patients' quality of life and survival. The progressive weakness of the respiratory muscles, including the diaphragm, is central to pulmonary function deterioration, resulting in a series of respiratory complications that eventually lead to respiratory failure, the primary cause of death among patients with ALS [9].

Initially, diaphragm weakness compromises thoracic excursion and forced vital capacity (FVC), one of the primary parameters used to monitor respiratory function. The diaphragm, which is responsible for most inspiration, when weakened, limits the expansion of the thoracic cavity, resulting in decreased lung volumes. As the disease advances, accessory respiratory muscles, including the intercostals and neck muscles, may become increasingly engaged. However, this compensation is temporary and insufficient to maintain adequate ventilation in the long term [10].

As diaphragmatic dysfunction worsens, the phenomenon of paradoxical abdominal movement is observed, where, during inhalation, the dysfunctional diaphragm is drawn inward into the thoracic cavity instead of moving downward. This clinical sign indicates severe respiratory weakness and is associated with a significant reduction in FVC and thoracic excursion. The resulting hypoventilation leads to hypercapnia and hypoxemia, exacerbating the sensation of dyspnea, especially during sleep, and increasing the risk of complications such as aspiration pneumonia and lung infections, including pneumonia [1].

Assessing pulmonary function is essential from the first signs of muscle weakness in patients with ALS. Measurements such as FVC and slow vital capacity (SVC) are used to predict the progression of respiratory dysfunction and survival. Studies show that FVC, especially when measured in the supine position, is a sensitive marker for detecting early diaphragmatic weakness. Moreover, SVC has proven to be an important predictor of survival and is correlated with disease progression, particularly in patients with bulbar onset or respiratory involvement [11].

The progression of respiratory weakness in ALS not only worsens dyspnea and exercise intolerance but also interferes with the ability to cough and clear secretions, increasing the risk of severe respiratory infections. Respiratory failure, made worse by diaphragmatic dysfunction and weakness of the accessory muscles, becomes a medical emergency as the disease advances, requiring interventions such as NIV or, in more severe cases, tracheostomy [11].

Early and continuous assessment of respiratory function is fundamental for effective disease management, helping to improve patients' quality of life and survival. By understanding how to manage these complexities, more targeted and effective therapeutic approaches can be developed, providing more humanized care focusing on the specific needs of each ALS patient [12].

Respiratory changes associated with disease progression can cause impairment of the upper airways, including the pharynx, larynx, and oral cavity. These are critical components for speech and swallowing. These processes depend on the complex coordination of various muscle groups, many of which are controlled by motor neurons that are progressively affected in ALS. Motor neuron degeneration results in muscle weakness, dysarthria (difficulty articulating speech), and dysphagia (difficulty swallowing) [12].

Dysarthria in patients with ALS occurs due to muscle weakness responsible for articulation, such as the tongue, lips, and soft palate. Speech production involves precise coordination between breathing and the muscle movements of the oral cavity, pharynx, and larynx. As ALS progresses, the ability to control these muscles diminishes, resulting in slurred, nasal, or unintelligible speech. Impairment of subglottic pressure, which is essential for voice modulation, further exacerbates these difficulties [11].

Dysphagia in ALS is a consequence of weakness in the muscles involved in swallowing, such as the tongue, pharyngeal, and esophageal muscles. Swallowing is a reflex process that involves multiple phases, including the oral, pharyngeal, and esophageal phases. Muscle weakness leads to difficulty initiating swallowing, reduces the effectiveness of food transport, and increases the risk of aspiration. Aspiration occurs when food or liquids enter the airways instead of going into the esophagus, heightening the risk of aspiration pneumonia, which is a common cause of mortality in patients with ALS [13].

These factors contribute to the overall decline in health and may accelerate disease progression. Speech impairment and swallowing are also directly related to the ventilatory pattern of patients. Studies indicate that the weakness of respiratory muscles, characteristic of ALS, reduces FVC and TV, negatively affecting the ability to speak and swallow. As the disease progresses, respiratory failure becomes a predominant concern, requiring interventions such as NIV, postural techniques, for instance leaning the head forward while swallowing, and modifications in food consistency to reduce the risk of aspiration [13].

4. Coughing and the need for strength in the laryngeal and respiratory muscles

Coughing is a fundamental defense mechanism of the respiratory system, designed to protect the airways from excessive secretions, irritants, and foreign bodies. To be effective, coughing depends on the precise coordination of the respiratory and laryngeal muscles [14]. This section explores the physiology of coughing, emphasizing the critical need for adequate muscular strength to ensure its efficacy, particularly in conditions such as ALS, where muscle weakness significantly compromises this vital function.

4.1 Physiology of coughing

Coughing is a reflex response that can be voluntary or involuntary, initiated by stimuli in the airway receptors. The coughing process can be divided into three main phases (**Figure 2**) [14]:

1. *Inspiratory phase*: this begins with a deep inhalation, increasing lung volume and preparing the respiratory system to generate the pressure needed for expulsion.

DOI: http://dx.doi.org/10.5772/intechopen.1007751

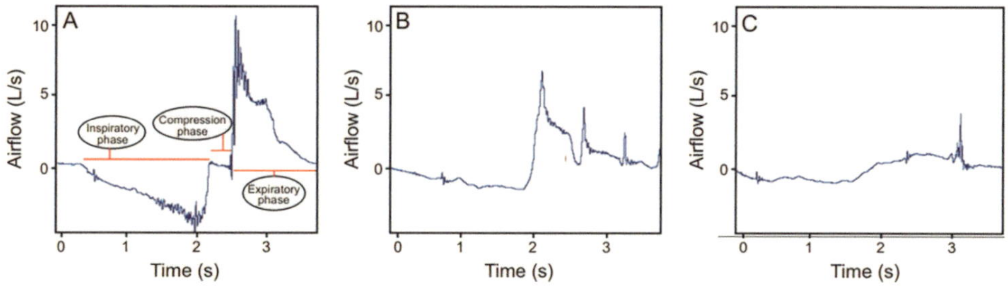

Figure 2.
Representation of spirometry during voluntary coughing.

2. *Compressive phase*: the glottis closes briefly to allow an increase in intrathoracic pressure.

3. *Expulsive phase*: the abrupt opening of the glottis results in an explosive expulsion of air from the lungs, carrying away secretions or irritating particles. The speed and flow of the expiratory air are crucial for the effectiveness of the cough, which is directly influenced by the strength of the muscles involved.

Spirometry waveform during voluntary coughing representing A: cough flow with distinct inspiratory and expiratory parameters in a healthy individual, illustrating the three phases of coughing from which the objective temporal airflow parameters are computed and aberrant. Cough flow in two individuals with ALS: B: spinal onset and C: bulbar onset. Source: Adapted from Andersen et al. [14].

The laryngeal muscles play a central role in modulating airflow during coughing. During the compressive phase, the larynx needs to quickly close the glottis to allow for the accumulation of intrathoracic pressure. This requires efficient contraction of the laryngeal muscles, such as the cricothyroid, which adjusts the tension of the vocal cords, and the thyroarytenoid, which controls glottic closure [15].

The strength of the laryngeal muscles is crucial for achieving a rapid and effective glottal closure. Any impairment in the function of these muscles, as seen in neuromuscular diseases (NMDs), can lead to inadequate glottal closure, resulting in a weak cough that is unable to effectively expel material from the airways. The respiratory muscles, including the diaphragm, intercostals, and abdominals, are responsible for generating the necessary pressure for the expulsive phase of the cough. These muscles must contract with sufficient force to increase intrathoracic pressure, which is the driving force behind the expiratory airflow during coughing [15].

4.2 Impact of muscle weakness on cough

The weakness of the laryngeal and respiratory muscles compromises all aspects of coughing. In patients with ALS, motor neuron degeneration results in the progressive weakness of these muscles, which manifests as a weak and ineffective cough. The inability to generate adequate expiratory airflow means that patients cannot clear secretions from the airways, increasing the risk of pulmonary infections and asphyxiation [16].

Weakness in coughing can lead to severe complications, including recurrent pneumonia and atelectasis (lung collapse), which are common in individuals with ALS. The ineffectiveness of coughing also contributes to the retention of carbon dioxide (hypercapnia) and hypoxia, further exacerbating respiratory failure [16].

4.3 Strategies to improve muscle strength and coughing

Considering the critical role of the laryngeal and respiratory muscles in coughing, several strategies can be implemented to improve cough effectiveness in patients with muscle weakness [13]:

1. *Respiratory exercises*: targeted exercises to strengthen the laryngeal and respiratory muscles can be implemented. Therapy may include diaphragmatic breathing techniques, respiratory resistance exercises, and specific training for the laryngeal muscles [13].

2. *Cough assistance*: cough assistance devices, such as mechanical insufflation-exsufflation devices, can be used to help patients who cannot generate an effective cough on their own. These devices apply positive pressure to the airways during inspiration and negative pressure during expiration, simulating the cough process and helping to clear secretions.

3. *Noninvasive ventilation (NIV)*: NIV can be used to improve ventilation and intrathoracic pressure, facilitating a more effective cough. In some cases, it may be combined with cough assistance to maximize secretion clearance.

4. *Breath stacking*: this technique involves introducing successive volumes of air into the lungs before attempting a cough, thereby increasing the total lung volume and the intrathoracic pressure available for expulsion during coughing.

5. Expiratory muscle training (EMT) to improve coughing in ALS

EMT is a promising intervention to improve expiratory function by increasing the subglottic pressure necessary for effective coughing and airway protection. It focuses on strengthening the muscles responsible for expiration, such as the abdominal and intercostal muscles, generating higher expiratory pressures. In individuals with ALS, weakness of these muscles can lead to ineffective coughing, increasing the risk of respiratory complications [17].

Clinical studies have shown that EMT is a viable and effective intervention for improving respiratory function in ALS. In a study conducted by Plowman et al. [17], the feasibility and impact of EMT on expiratory force generation capacity, swallowing kinematics, cough physiology, and airway protection were evaluated in individuals with ALS. The results indicated that EMT was safe and well-tolerated and led to immediate improvements in expiratory force and hyoid movement during swallowing. The hyoid movement is a crucial event in swallowing, as it facilitates the relaxation and opening of the upper esophageal sphincter, allowing the effective transit of the food bolus from the pharynx to the esophagus and reducing the risk of aspiration.

Another study conducted by Plowman et al. [18] investigated the effect of a 5-week EMT program in individuals with ALS and found significant improvements in respiratory and bulbar function. Although there were no statistically significant differences in cough spirometry measurements, the 22% reduction in the inspiratory phase suggests a clinical improvement in the ability to inflate the lungs efficiently and in glottic closure, both of which are essential for producing an effective cough.

5.1 EMT techniques to improve outcomes

EMT can be complemented by other respiratory techniques, such as breath stacking. This technique involves accumulating successive volumes of air in the lungs before attempting to cough, thereby increasing the inspired volume and, consequently, the peak cough flow. The increase in inspired volume can enhance the effectiveness of EMT, helping clear secretions and prevent atelectasis. Furthermore, combining EMT with inspiratory muscle training can provide a more comprehensive approach to respiratory rehabilitation in patients with ALS, improving both expiratory and inspiratory pressures, resulting in a more robust overall respiratory function.

Maintaining the ability to generate adequate subglottic pressure is vital for the quality of life of patients with ALS. A study by Plowman et al. [18] demonstrated that EMT, when performed over 12 weeks, had a positive impact on specific respiratory capacity and airway clearance functions during the early stages of ALS. These results suggest that EMT not only improves respiratory function but may also have a positive effect on patient survival.

Although EMT has shown promising results, further research is needed to determine the optimal training intensity, resistance load specifications, and potential long-term benefits. Further studies are needed to explore how combining EMT with other respiratory techniques, such as breath stacking, can optimize clinical outcomes [19].

The rapid progression of ALS and the variation in treatment response among individuals highlight the importance of personalizing therapeutic interventions. Integrating EMT into a comprehensive respiratory rehabilitation plan can provide significant benefits for patients, helping to preserve respiratory function and prolong survival.

6. Volumetric recruitment and impact on the upper airway

Forced expiration plays a crucial role in clearing the lungs, trachea, and larynx. Throat clearing involves the closure of the supraglottic folds, effectively moving material from the laryngeal vestibule to the pharynx. The hawking technique involves a rapid exhalation combined with the soft palate making contact with the base of the tongue. This action is used to move material from the oropharynx to the front of the mouth. Furthermore, postswallowing is an important airway protection behavior, preventing the entry of fluids, food, or secretions into the larynx and lungs.

The supraglottic swallowing maneuver aims for the voluntary closure of the vocal folds before and during swallowing, causing the arytenoid cartilage to tilt toward the base of the epiglottis. This technique is especially recommended to improve two of the most common swallowing challenges faced by people with ALS [20].

Clinical guidelines recommend daily pulmonary volume recruitment (PVR) therapy to combat the decline in lung volume through assisted inflation [21]. PVR is a technique often used by individuals with NMDs to achieve higher lung volumes and improve coughing. This technique involves providing consecutive "breaths" with

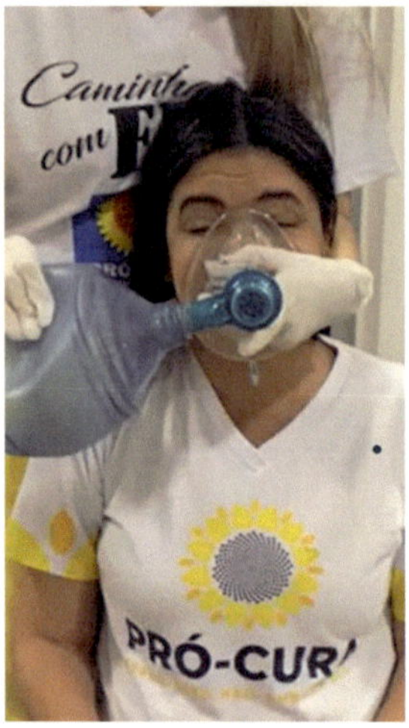

Figure 3.
Individual performing pulmonary volume recruitment. Source: Personal archive (authorized by the individual).

inspiratory pressure to the airways, using a manual self-inflating bag, with or without a unidirectional valve, connected to an oronasal mask or mouthpiece (**Figure 3**). The assisted breaths accumulate, resulting in a greater pulmonary inflation volume than can be achieved with spontaneous breathing. Previous research has shown that PVR increases maximum inspiratory capacity (MIC) or pulmonary inflation capacity (PIC), as well as the peak expiratory flow during the maneuver. Retrospective and cohort studies in NMDs suggest that PVR may slow lung function decline [21].

The PVR, also known as breath stacking, is a simple, low-cost manual inflation technique that enhances coughing. Breath stacking maneuvers are essential for maintaining lung capacity and facilitating expulsion in patients with neuromuscular disorders, especially in children [22]. In adults, using an inflation bag with a unidirectional valve increases lung volume. In ALS, breath stacking and MIC are fundamental methods for improving cough effectiveness and providing muscular rest [23, 24]. These techniques rely on good muscular strength in the oropharynx, glottis, and larynx [22].

Although progressive muscle weakness is a central characteristic of ALS, using strength-focused interventions has historically been discouraged due to the concern of muscle overload, which could accelerate physical decline. Traditionally, treatment models for ALS have been primarily palliative in nature. However, recent evidence indicates that light to moderate exercise programs, started early, can enhance physiological capacity and strength, prevent disuse atrophy and deconditioning, as well as alleviate pain and spasticity, and improve the overall psychological well-being of individuals with ALS [25].

7. Perspectives on muscle training in neuromuscular diseases

Integrating expiratory muscle training (EMT) with other respiratory rehabilitation strategies can maximize clinical benefits, providing a valuable intervention to improve respiratory function and survival in ALS. Studies [26, 27] on respiratory muscle strength training interventions in individuals with ALS have shown transient improvements in inspiratory and expiratory pressures, although long-term effects are still inconclusive. Plowman [28] observed that these interventions resulted in transient gains in variables such as maximum inspiratory pressures and respiratory benefits on the Amyotrophic Lateral Sclerosis Functional Rating Scale (ALSFRS), but the effects were not considered significant.

Clinical trials [27, 28] demonstrate that inspiratory and expiratory muscle strength training programs can extend survival by up to 14 months and improve respiratory and bulbar function, serving as potential prognostic indicators of survival. However, the need for control groups and further investigation is crucial to validate these hypotheses.

Techniques such as breath stacking and EMT have proven viable, safe, and beneficial in enhancing expiratory force generation, swallowing function, and airway protection, especially in early stages of ALS [17]. Moreover, increased inspired volume through breath stacking can lead to improvements in both reflexive and voluntary cough, aiding in mucus clearance and preventing atelectasis.

The recent study by Plowman et al. [19] suggests that respiratory training interventions may positively impact the physiological capacity of respiration and airway clearance function in the early stages of the disease. However, they emphasize the need for additional studies to determine the ideal intensity and long-term benefits. Short-duration training, such as the 8-week protocol applied by Tabor et al. [6], also demonstrated promising results, including increased peak cough flow and expiratory muscle strength.

In 2020, Dorça et al. [29] conducted a pilot study involving 8 patients with ALS who followed a set of techniques combining pulmonary recruitment with expiratory resistance exercise, called respiratory readaptation and reorganization therapy (TR3). This therapy consists of a series of three respiratory exercises, including maximum lung inflation using an inflation bag (pulmonary recruitment) and slow, gradual expiratory muscle training (endurance training). The study described the technique and demonstrated its impact on the airway during its execution. A notable aspect of the study was the innovative use of videofluoroscopy to demonstrate the techniques (**Figure 4**).

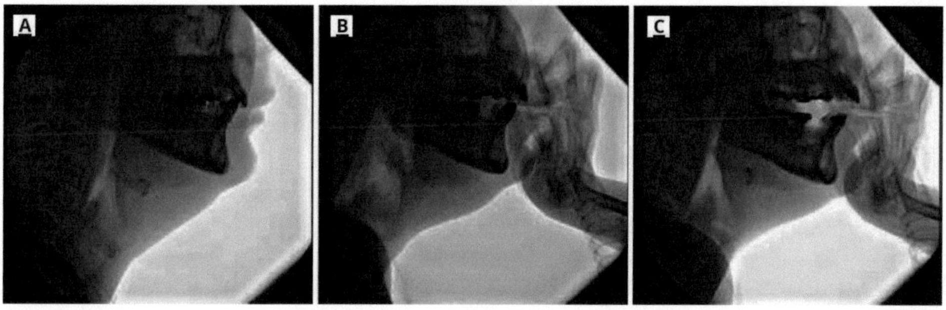

Figure 4.
Impact of Volumetric Recruitment against Expiratory Resistance. Details of the main videofluoroscopic photos of interest analyzed. Overview of the differences in the pharyngeal constriction area during rest and during respiratory training. A. Resting position showing measurements of the pharyngeal area; B. Example of maximum pharyngeal expansion (MPE) during the technique with positive unidirectional pressure valve (PUPV); C. Maximum pharyngeal constriction (MPC) during the PUPV technique. Source: Dorça et al. [29].

8. Conclusion

Understanding the factors related to respiratory dysfunction in NMDs, specifically ALS, is essential for prescribing individualized therapeutic approaches aimed at slowing the progression of the disease. EMT is a systematic technique with promising prospects for exercise prescriptions in this population. However, studies with more robust methodologies, such as clinical trials and control groups, are required for a better understanding of the effects of this therapy and its impact on NMDs.

Author details

Alessandra Carneiro Dorça[1*] and Letícia de Araújo Morais[2]

1 Integrated Training and Advanced Studies Center (CEAFI), Alessandra Dorça Institute, Goiânia, GO, Brazil

2 Estácio de Sá University Center in Goiás, Goiânia, GO, Brazil

*Address all correspondence to: diretoria.comercial@ceafi.com.br

References

[1] Patel N, Chong K, Baydur A. Methods and applications in respiratory physiology: Respiratory mechanics, drive and muscle function in neuromuscular and chest wall disorders. Frontiers in Physiology. 2022;**13**:838414. DOI: 10.3389/fphys.2022.838414

[2] Ravits JM, La Spada AR. ALS motor phenotype heterogeneity, focality, and spread: Deconstructing motor neuron degeneration. Neurology. 2009;**73**(10):805-811. DOI: 10.1212/WNL.0b013e3181b6bbbd

[3] Tomik B, Guiloff R. Dysarthria in amyotrophic lateral sclerosis: A review. Amyotrophic Lateral Sclerosis. 2010;**11**(1-2):4-15

[4] Nichols NL, Van Dyke J, Nashold L, Satriotomo I, Suzuki M, Mitchell GS. Ventilatory control in ALS. Respiratory Physiology & Neurobiology. 2013;**189**(2):429-437. DOI: 10.1016/j.resp.2013.05.016. Epub 2013 May 18

[5] Bach JR, Alba AS, Saporito LR. Intermittent positive pressure ventilation via the mouth as an alternative to tracheostomy for 257 ventilator users. Chest. 1993;**103**(1):174-182. DOI: 10.1378/chest.103.1.174

[6] Tabor LC, Rosado KM, Robison R, Hegland K, Humbert IA, Plowman EK. Respiratory training in an individual with amyotrophic lateral sclerosis. Annals of Clinical Translational Neurology. 2016;**3**(10):819-823. DOI: 10.1002/acn3.342

[7] Quinn C, Elman L. Amyotrophic lateral sclerosis and other motor neuron diseases. Continuum (Minneap Minn). 2020;**26**(5):1323-1347. DOI: 10.1212/CON.0000000000000911

[8] Sheers NL, Berlowitz DJ, Dirago RK, Naughton P, Henderson S, Rigoni A, et al. Rapidly and slowly progressive neuromuscular disease: Differences in pulmonary function, respiratory tract infections and response to lung volume recruitment therapy (LVR). BMJ Open Respiratory Research. 2022;**9**(1):e001241. DOI: 10.1136/bmjresp-2022-001241

[9] Hardiman O, Al-Chalabi A, Chio A, Corr EM, Logroscino G, Robberecht W, et al. Amyotrophic lateral sclerosis. Nature Reviews. Disease Primers. 2017;**3**:17071. DOI: 10.1038/nrdp.2017.71. Erratum in: Nat Rev Dis Primers 2017 Oct 20;3:17085. doi: 10.1038/nrdp.2017.85

[10] Iguchi N, Mano T, Iwasa N, Ozaki M, Yamada N, Kikutsuji N, et al. Thoracic excursion is a biomarker for evaluating respiratory function in amyotrophic lateral sclerosis. Frontiers in Neurology. 2022;**13**:853469. DOI: 10.3389/fneur.2022.853469

[11] Huang X, Du C, Yang Q, Fan D. Comparison of slow and forced vital capacity on ability to evaluate respiratory function in bulbar-involved amyotrophic lateral sclerosis. Frontiers in Neurology. 2022;**13**:938256. DOI: 10.3389/fneur.2022.938256

[12] Niedermeyer S, Murn M, Choi PJ. Respiratory failure in amyotrophic lateral sclerosis. Chest. 2019;**155**(2):401-408. DOI: 10.1016/j.chest.2018.06.035. Epub 2018 Jul 7

[13] Chatwin M, Toussaint M, Gonçalves MR, Sheers N, Mellies U, Gonzales-Bermejo J, et al. Airway clearance techniques in neuromuscular disorders: A state of the art review. Respiratory Medicine. 2018;**136**:98-110. DOI: 10.1016/j.rmed.2018.01.012. Epub 2018 Feb 6

[14] Andersen TM, Hov B, Halvorsen T, Røksund OD, Vollsæter M. Upper airway assessment and responses during mechanically assisted cough. Respiratory Care. 2021;**66**(7):1196-1213. DOI: 10.4187/respcare.08960. Epub 2021 Feb 12

[15] Andersen TM, Halvorsen T, Fondenes O, Heimdal JH, Røksund OD, Vollsæter M, et al. Larynx: The complex gateway to the lungs. Respiratory Care. 2019;**64**(7):866-869. DOI: 10.4187/respcare.06989

[16] Tabor-Gray LC, Gallestagui A, Vasilopoulos T, Plowman EK. Characteristics of impaired voluntary cough function in individuals with amyotrophic lateral sclerosis. Amyotrophic Lateral Sclerosis and Frontotemporal Degeneration. 2019;**20**(1-2):37-42. DOI: 10.1080/21678421.2018.1510011. Epub 2019 Jan 17

[17] Plowman EK, Watts SA, Tabor L, Robison R, Gaziano J, Domer AS, et al. Impact of expiratory strength training in amyotrophic lateral sclerosis. Muscle & Nerve. 2016;**54**(1):48-53. DOI: 10.1002/mus.24990. Epub 2016 Mar 3

[18] Plowman EK, Tabor-Gray L, Rosado KM, Vasilopoulos T, Robison R, Chapin JL, et al. Impact of expiratory strength training in amyotrophic lateral sclerosis: Results of a randomized, sham-controlled trial. Muscle & Nerve. 2019;**59**(1):40-46. DOI: 10.1002/mus.26292. Epub 2018 Nov 29

[19] Plowman EK, Gray LT, Chapin J, Anderson A, Vasilopoulos T, Gooch C, et al. Respiratory strength training in amyotrophic lateral sclerosis: A double-blind, randomized, multicenter, sham-controlled trial. Neurology. 2023;**100**(15):e1634-e1642. DOI: 10.1212/WNL.0000000000206830. Epub 2023 Feb 20

[20] McCool FD, Rosen MJ. Nonpharmacologic airway clearance therapies: ACCP evidence-based clinical practice guidelines. Chest. 2006;**129**(1 Suppl):250S-259S. DOI: 10.1378/chest.129.1_suppl.250S

[21] Sheers NL, O'Sullivan R, Howard ME, Berlowitz DJ. The role of lung volume recruitment therapy in neuromuscular disease: A narrative review. Frontiers in Rehabilitation Sciences. 2023;**4**:1164628. DOI: 10.3389/fresc.2023.1164628

[22] Bach J. Air stacking for cough assistance. Muscle & Nerve. 2004;**30**(5):680-681. DOI: 10.1002/mus.20116. author reply 681

[23] Jenkins HM, Stocki A, Kriellaars D, Pasterkamp H. Breath stacking in children with neuromuscular disorders. Pediatric Pulmonology. 2014;**49**(6):544-553. DOI: 10.1002/ppul.22865. Epub 2013 Aug 16

[24] Barcelar Jde M, Aliverti A, Rattes C, Ximenes ME, Campos SL, Brandão DC, et al. The expansion of the pulmonary rib cage during breath stacking is influenced by age in obese women. PLoS One. 2014;**9**(11):e110959. DOI: 10.1371/journal.pone.0110959

[25] Dal Bello-Haas V, Florence JM. Therapeutic exercise for people with amyotrophic lateral sclerosis or motor neuron disease. Cochrane Database of Systematic Reviews. 2013;**2013**(5):CD005229. DOI: 10.1002/14651858.CD005229.pub3

[26] Cheah BC, Boland RA, Brodaty NE, Zoing MC, Jeffery SE, McKenzie DK, et al. INSPIRATIonAL--INSPIRAtory muscle training in amyotrophic lateral sclerosis. Amyotrophic Lateral Sclerosis. 2009;**10**(5-6):384-392. DOI: 10.3109/17482960903082218

[27] Pinto S, Swash M, de Carvalho M. Respiratory exercise in amyotrophic lateral sclerosis. Amyotrophic Lateral Sclerosis. 2012;**13**(1):33-43. DOI: 10.3109/17482968.2011.626052

[28] Plowman EK. Is there a role for exercise in the management of bulbar dysfunction in amyotrophic lateral sclerosis? Journal of Speech, Language, and Hearing Research. 2015;**58**(4):1151-1166. DOI: 10.1044/2015_JSLHR-S-14-0270

[29] Dorça A, Alcântara LA, Diniz DS, Sarmet M, Menezes Mateus SR, Franco Oliveira LV, et al. Comparison between breath stacking technique associated with expiratory muscle training and breath stacking technique in amyotrophic lateral sclerosis patients: Protocol for randomized single blind trial. Contemporary Clinical Trials Communications. 2020;**19**:100647. DOI: 10.1016/j.conctc.2020.100647

Chapter 4

Approach to Peripheral Neuropathy

Chee Shin Yong and Mathew Alexander

Abstract

Peripheral neuropathy is frequently encountered in the clinical setting by doctors of various specialties. Neuropathies can be approached based on the temporal profile, spatial pattern and pathology. There is a need for eliciting a focused history, co-morbidities, exposure to medications and toxins, family history and examination, electrodiagnostic testing and laboratory testing. The prevalence of neuropathy is based on epidemiological studies, and it is important to know the yield of etiological diagnosis, even after extensive investigations. Acute neuropathies include Guillain-Barre syndrome, porphyria, ICU-acquired paresis, neuropathies associated with systemic diseases, autoimmune diseases, nutritional, toxic and genetic disorders. It's important to have knowledge about electro-diagnostic characteristics, the role of nerve biopsy in select cases, treatment, both disease-modifying and symptomatic and outcome.

Keywords: peripheral neuropathy, prevalence, temporal profile, spatial, electromyoneurography, pathology, treatment, outcomes

1. Introduction

The peripheral nervous system consists of all nerves distal to the spinal cord including motor neurons that originate in the spinal cord, the sensory nerves that terminate in the spinal cord, as well as autonomic nerve fibers. Peripheral neuropathy is the disorder of the said system and is one of the most common neurological presentations. Peripheral neuropathy is commonly encountered and is seen in several disorders like metabolic syndrome, diabetes mellitus, uremia, infections, parainfectious, paraproteinemic, nutritional, toxins and inherited causes. Peripheral neuropathy affects all populations worldwide, with prevalence increasing with age, with over half the cases being attributed to diabetes after work up by a neurologist. The International Diabetes Federation estimates 425 million people worldwide have diabetes, which makes it a large global epidemic, and the most prevalent complication is neuropathy, distal symmetric sensory neuropathy being most common. About 12% of global expenditure or $ 727 billion is directed to diabetes and its complications.

The prevalence of peripheral neuropathy based on several population-based studies is estimated to be between 2.4 per 100,000 with prevalence increasing with age and 8/100000, with diabetes being the most common cause [1, 2].

Diagnosis of peripheral neuropathy could be quite challenging, given the spectrum, heterogeneous presentation and diverse etiology. It is vital to have a structured approach with respect to eliciting a good history and clinical examination to elucidate the temporal profile, spatial pattern, fiber type and underlying pathogenesis and do appropriate investigations.

Identifying features of time-sensitive treatable causes of peripheral neuropathy is crucial to limit nerve damage and avoid poor outcome. Screening of asymptomatic patients at risk of peripheral neuropathy secondary to systemic diseases is vital to avoid complications. Despite extensive investigations, in up to 30% of patients, no cause can yet be identified [3, 4].

2. Step 1: First and foremost, is there a peripheral neuropathy?

It is prudent to exclude cortical and spinal involvement. Hyperreflexia and spasticity would favor localization to a central pathology. If signs and symptoms do not localize to either central or peripheral nervous systems, psychogenic factors need to be considered. Most presenting complaints are more sensory, as motor and autonomic dysfunctions are usually not apparent to the patient immediately. Further inquiry of dry skin, cracked heels, postural dizziness and erectile dysfunction will need to be made (**Table 1**).

Symptoms	Positive	Negative
Sensory	Paraesthesia Burning, electric-like, hypersensitivity, squeezing/tightness	Numbness Reduced sensation Unsteadiness
Motor	Cramps, fasciculations	Weakness Atrophy

Table 1.
The sensory and motor symptoms and signs found in peripheral neuropathy.

3. Step 2: Spatial involvement/distribution – Which part of the peripheral nervous system is involved and to which extent?

The peripheral nervous system is composed of somatic (sensory and motor) and autonomic nerves. Sensory cell bodies are in dorsal root ganglion or one of the sensory ganglia of sensory cranial nerves. A motor unit consist of anterior horn cell, its axon, the neuromuscular junction and the muscle fiber it innervates. Autonomic nerves are composed of two neuron pathways (preganglionic or postganglionic) and have parasympathetic and sympathetic arm.

On looking at the spatial pattern, there could be one nerve, several discrete nerves or multiple nerves diffusely involved:

- Mononeuropathy
- Mononeuropathy multiplex
- Distal-predominant polyneuropathy

- Distal and proximal polyneuropathy
- Plexopathy
- Radiculopathy
- Asymmetric – unusual

Length-dependent neuropathies start symmetrically with sensory disturbance in the feet and, as it ascends to the knee, then involves finger tips and then forearms, and this is a dying back neuropathy. Immune-mediated neuropathies like GBS and CIDP have a non-length-dependent pattern and have proximal predominant weakness and trunk weakness. Neuropathy that begins in one leg or hands indicates an asymmetric disorder, and a careful history is vital as over a period this becomes confluent and looks symmetrical. Careful examination helps in discerning asymmetries in the degree of nerve involvement. Mononeuritis multiplex could be due to vasculitis, leprosy, CIDP variants and multifocal motor neuropathy with conduction block. The neuropathy in lepromatous neuropathy has a temperature-dependent distribution affecting superficial often unnamed nerves from the coolest regions of body, ear lobes, nose and dorsal extremities.

Nerve conduction studies and needle electromyography help in confirming the presence of spatial distribution and help in ascertaining nerve-muscle continuity and assess the extent of denervation/re-innervation [5, 6].

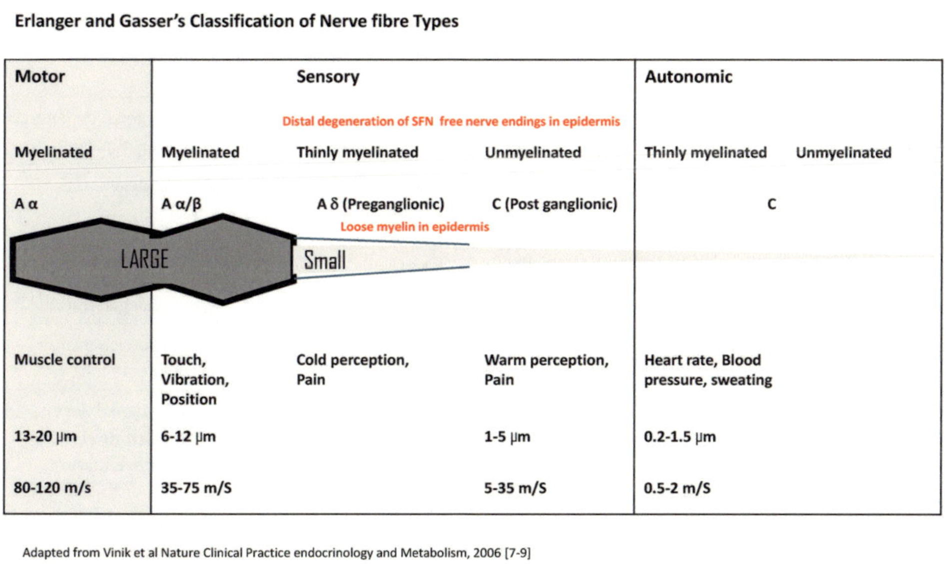

Figure 1.
Classification of nerve fiber types. Adapted from [7–9].

4. Step 3: What nerve fibers are involved?

Large fiber nerves include motor nerves, A-alpha and A-Beta sensory nerves. [Erlanger/Gasser classification] Small fiber nerves include A-delta that respond to pressure-producing sensation of fast pain and C-fibers that mediate pain and temperature. Smaller fibers are preferentially affected in systemic disorders and are length dependent with longest and most distal nerves affected first (lower limbs). Autonomic nerves are unmyelinated and outnumber somatic nerves (**Figure 1**).

5. Step 4: Temporal profile

When one looks at the temporal profile, acute neuropathies occur within 4 weeks, subacute neuropathies occur within 4–8 weeks and chronic neuropathies, beyond 8 weeks. Most acquired causes are acute to subacute while hereditary neuropathies are chronic (**Table 2**) [6].

Types	Main etiological groups	Sub-classification	Pathology
Primary	Guillain-Barre Syndrome	Acute Inflammatory Demyelinating Polyneuropathy (AIDP)	Demyelination (± conduction block) with variable axonal loss
		Acute Motor Axonal Neuropathy (AMAN)	
			Axonal degeneration of motor fibers
		Acute Motor and Sensory Axonal Polyneuropathy (AMSAN)	
			Axonal degeneration of motor and sensory fibers
		Miller Fisher Syndrome	
			Mixed axonal degeneration and demyelination
Secondary	Autoimmune and malignant disorders	Connective tissue diseases, Poly-Arteritis Nodosa, Wegener's granulomatosis, Systemic Lupus Erythematosus, rheumatoid arthritis, Sjogren's, cancer	Axonal degeneration
	Infectious disease	AIDS, neuroboreliosis, Hepatitis C	Axonal degeneration
	Metabolic disorders	Diabetes Mellitus; Uremia; Acute Porphyria; Critical Illness Neuropathy*	Axonal degeneration
	Toxins	Arsenic, Amiodarone, Vincristine, Cisplastin, Pyridoxine, Disulfram, Gold salts, Glue, Alcohol, Organophosphates	Mostly axonal degeneration (Amiodarone associated with demyelination

**Standard Textbooks do not mention CIN in the Classification of Acute Neuropathy.*

Table 2.
Classification of acute polyneuropathy.

6. Step 5: Are there other associated features?

Physical features: It's important to look for associated features like alopecia, madarosis, corneal opacities, Bitot's spots, scleritis/episcleritis, malar rash, angular stomatitis, cheilitis, blue line on gums, Mees' lines, cutaneous nerve thickening, pes cavus and hammer toes (**Figure 2**).

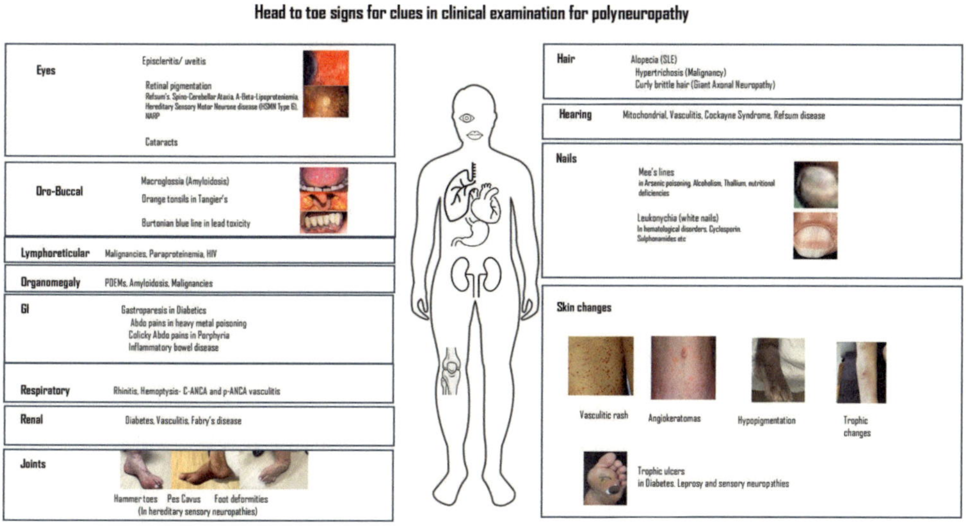

Figure 2.
Mini atlas on head-to-toe clinical signs in clinical examination for polyneuropathy.

7. Step 6: Axonal versus demyelinating

Many neuropathies have overlapping pathological features, but it is important to define the predominant pathophysiological damage. Demyelination affects large, myelinated fibers causing reduced conduction velocities. There would be manifestation of motor weakness, paraesthesia and absent deep tendon reflexes. A hallmark for acquired demyelinating neuropathies is severe motor weakness with minimal atrophy. They are symmetric but, early into illness, could be asymmetric. Damage to myelin sheath is repaired by Schwann cells in 6–12 weeks.

Damage to axon (microtubules and microfilaments) affects smaller fibers particularly the smaller fibers at the most distal part first presenting as dying back phenomenon. This manifests as muscle wasting along with weakness. Nerve conduction studies and EMG are required to delineate the pathophysiology. In small fiber neuropathies, it might be prudent to do sympathetic skin responses and cardiovascular autonomic function tests, and the physician might need epidermal biopsies to look at epidermal nerve fiber density [10–13].

8. Medical and social conditions: Alcohol, diets, occupational exposure

After ascertaining the neuropathy, the physician needs to review all the systems, perform meticulous examination and look for an underlying medical disorder. Diabetes mellitus, connective tissue disease, underlying infection, cancer, malnutrition, and exposure to drugs, alcohol or occupational exposure to toxins need to be considered and addressed [12–15].

9. Family history

Inherited neuropathies are detected in 40% of undiagnosed neuropathies in dedicated centres. The diagnosis could remain elusive due to reasons such as inability to elicit a family history, occurrence of de-novo mutations (PMP gene 22 gene duplication), recessive and X-linked recessive mutations, and the neuropathy could remain asymptomatic for decades. These patients could have signs of neuropathy with skeletal markers like pes cavus or kyphoscoliosis but could be unaware because of slow progression. A careful history to elicit the inheritance pattern, clinical examination and nerve conduction studies will help to guide genetic tests. The most common types are CMT 1A, CMT1B, CMTX and HNPP. There could be situations in which family history is lacking, with atypical presentation like CIDP mimics. Knowledge on the phenotypes of various inherited neuropathies is required for genetic counseling [16–18].

10. Tying it together

Having established neuropathy, there is a group where one might be able to establish a probable diagnosis like GBS and Diabetic Polyneuropathy. Another group where one could get clues from medical history and family history to help direct specific investigations. There could also be a group of chronic polyneuropathies where there are no defining feature or clue, and it is important to have a diagnostic algorithm for the said neuropathic syndrome.

11. Role of laboratory testing

It is important to focus and decide on further investigations. Basic laboratory investigations include a complete blood count, serum electrolytes, renal and liver function tests, screening for diabetes mellitus, immunofixation and immunoelectrophoresis. One must restrain from ordering a battery of laboratory tests and antibody panel without regard for the most probable cause of neuropathy [19, 20]. If there are no pointers to underlying cause, there needs to be judicious use of laboratory tests (**Table 3**).

Polyneuropathies	Investigations
Acute	Lumbar puncture/ CSF studies
	Ganglioside antibodies
	Urine/ fecal Porphyrins
	24 hr. urine for heavy metals (Arsenic, Thallium)
	Red cell Transketolase activity (Thiamine Deficient))
	Lyme Serology (Endemic Areas)
Subacute/ Chronic	Fasting glucose, HbA1C
	Serum Protein electrophoresis/ immune fixation
	HIV serology
	Vitamin B12 levels +/– Methylmalonic acid (MMA) levels
	Thyroid Function Tests
	Serum Triglycerides/ HDL (Tangier's disease)
	ANA, Anti-Ro, Anti-La

Table 3.
Recommended laboratory investigations for polyneuropathies.

11.1 Small fiber neuropathy

The symptoms are burning pain, allodynia, impaired pain and temperature sensations and the autonomic symptoms such as facial flushing, sicca, accommodation symptoms, hyper–/hypohidrosis, palpitations, orthostatic intolerance, gastroparesis, constipation, diarrhea and bladder disturbances. The etiology includes metabolic diseases (diabetes mellitus and hypothyroidism), drugs/toxins (e.g. alcohol, highly active anti-retroviral therapy (HAART), metronidazole and bortezomib), immune-mediated diseases (e.g. coeliac disease, Sjogren's syndrome and sarcoidosis) and paraneoplastic syndrome. Genetic causes include Fabry's disease, amyloidosis, SCN 9A and familial burning feet syndrome.

Investigations include sympathetic skin responses; cardiovascular autonomic function tests including RR interval on deep breathing and supine to standing; and beat to beat recording using Finometer for accurate non-invasive beat to beat recording, which could be used to differentiate orthostatic hypotension from postural tachycardia syndrome (**Tables 4** and **5**).

Immune Mediated Neuropathies- Autoantibodies associations with clinical phenotypes				
Disease	**Phenotype**	**Antigens**	**Antibody isotype**	**Clinical implications**
Acute Motor Axonal Neuropathy (AMAN)	Pure motor	GM1, M1b-GD1a	IgG	Guide to GBS subtype
		GD1a		
		GaINAc-GD1a		
Acute Motor and Sensory Axonal Neuropathy (AMSAN)	Motor and sensory	GM1 and GD1a	IgG	
Miller Fisher Syndrome	Ataxia, Ophthalmoplegia, Areflexia	GQ1b and GT1a	IgG	
Pharyngeal-Cervical-Brachial variant of GBS	Oropharyngeal, facial, neck and shoulder weakness	GT1, GQ1b and GD1a	IgG	
Multifocal Motor Neuropathy	Motor	GM1 and complex GM1:GaIC	IgM	Diagnostic guide
Chronic Inflammatory Demyelinating Polyneuroradiuclopathy (CIDP)	Aggressive onset and initial axonal involvement	Contactin 1	IgG4	Poor response to IV Ig
	Tremor, Ataxia and distal motor involvement	NF155	IgG4	
	Subacute onset, sensory Ataxia and conduction block	NF186 and NF140	IgG4	Good response to IV Ig and steroids

Adapted from [19].

Table 4.
Investigations for immune mediated neuropathies.

Small fiber polyneuropathy	Investigations
Acute	Fasting glucose, HbA1C
Subacute/Chronic	Fasting glucose, HbA1C
	ANA, anti-Ro, anti-La
	Serum Protein electrophoresis/ immune fixation
	Transthyretin Mutations
	Cholesterol/HDL (Tangier's disease)
	Leukocyte alpha galactosidase (Fabry's disease)

Table 5.
Recommended laboratory investigations for small fiber neuropathy.

12. Blood biomarkers of peripheral neuropathy

Neurophysiology is currently used as a biomarker, for both diagnostic and prognostic purposes. It has limitations due to the need for high skills, inter-operator variability and lack of sensitivity.

There has been development of ultrasensitive protein assays with a lower level of detection than that of traditional ELISA techniques. This has allowed markers of neuronal damage such as neurofilament light chains (NFL) to be accurately measured in blood. One of the key setbacks, however, is the inability to distinguish central from peripheral nerve damage. These biomarkers have been found to be effective at identifying patients with peripheral neuropathy compared to controls and show efficacy as a marker for disease activity in patients with rapidly progressive peripheral neuropathy such as vasculitis and amyloidosis. The use of axonal protein biomarkers like NFL in slowly progressive diseases with or without axonal loss such as Charcot-Marie-Tooth, CIDP and multifocal motor neuropathy is less certain. Measurements of relevant circulating micro-RNAs are showing great promise as the technology to quantify is well established and specific mRNAs could be identified for disease-specific states [21].

13. Genetic testing and algorithm

Nerve conduction studies would help guide what panel should be run for the most plausible etiology (**Figure 3**).

14. Role of imaging

Imaging has emerged to be a useful tool in investigating neuropathies and complements nerve conduction studies. The two modalities are nerve ultrasound and MRI including MR neurography, and in select cases, positron emission tomography is of value.

Nerve ultrasound is useful in evaluation of entrapment neuropathies, when NCS does not delineate and help in evaluating patients with CIDP and inherited neuropathies like HMSN. MRI including MR neurography is a useful tool to study brachial and lumbosacral plexopathies and could help in guiding fascicular biopsies [23–25].

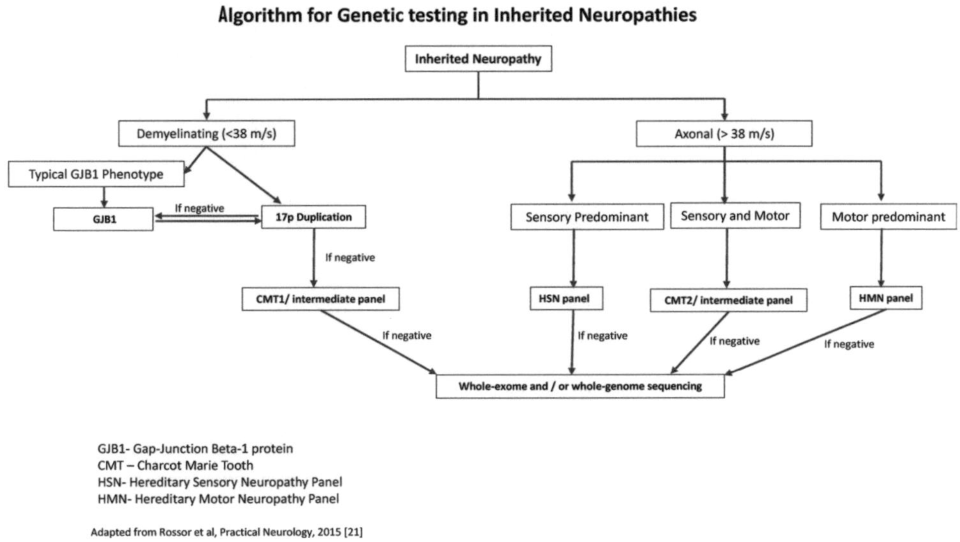

Figure 3.
Flow chart/algorithm for genetic testing in inherited neuropathies [22].

Included are examples of MR and ultrasound imaging in the evaluation of peripheral neuropathies and plexopathies (**Figures 4–9**).

14.1 Utility of nerve biopsy

Over recent years, though the utility of nerve biopsy has decreased, there is still a role in the diagnostic workup of neuropathies with definite indications such as in diagnosing vasculitis, leprosy, amyloidosis, sarcoidosis, Tangier and giant axonal neuropathy. It is important to consider the clinical setting, choose involved nerves and sometimes consider nerve-muscle-skin biopsies and the availability of appropriate neuropathological techniques. Sural nerve is preferred as it is purely sensory and accessible and in cases of non-systemic vasculitic neuropathy, superficial peroneal nerve or involved sensory nerves. Epidermal skin biopsy can also be performed for the diagnosis of small fiber neuropathy (**Figure 10**) [27].

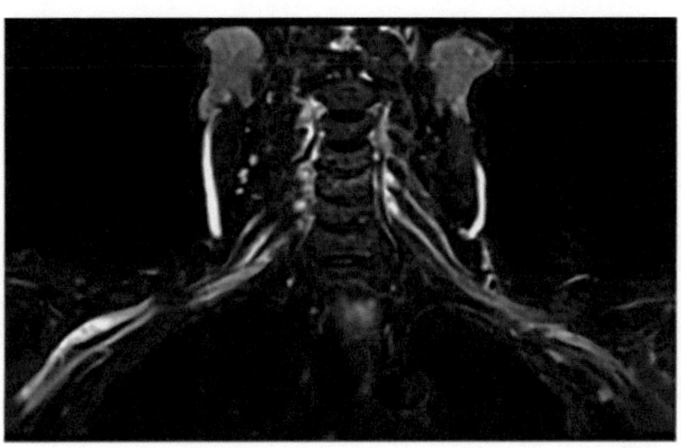

Figure 4.
MR Neurography showing thickened brachial plexus (bilateral) in a patient with CIDP [26].

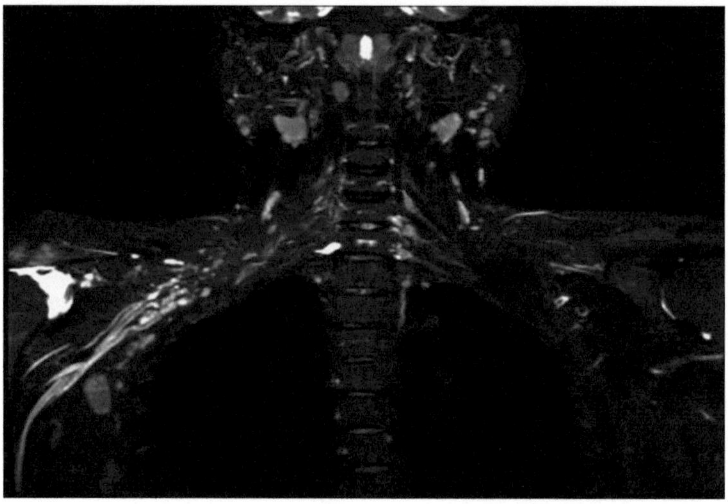

Figure 5.
Complete transection of preganglionic right brachial plexus with denervation atrophy of shoulder girdle muscles.

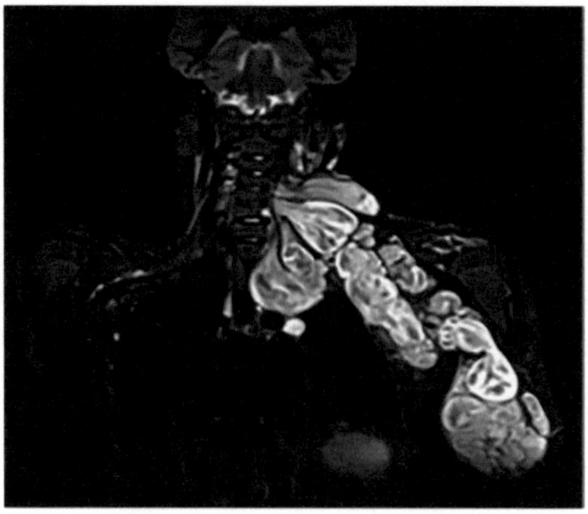

Figure 6.
Plexiform neurofibromatosis involving left brachial plexus.

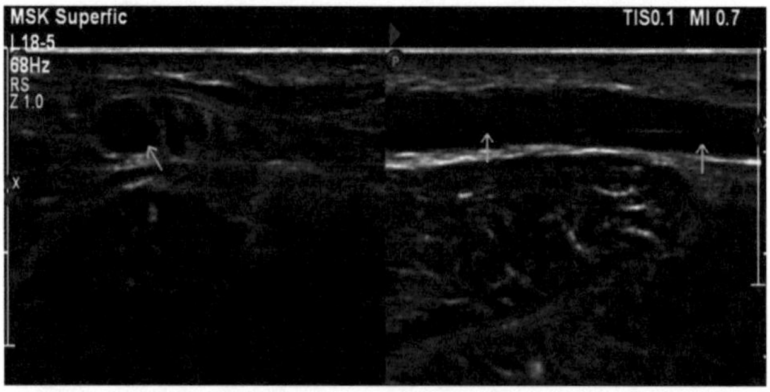

Figure 7.
Ultrasound images showing A: transverse and B: longitudinal images of common peroneal nerve with diffuse asymmetrical thickening of fascicles with preserved fascicular architecture.

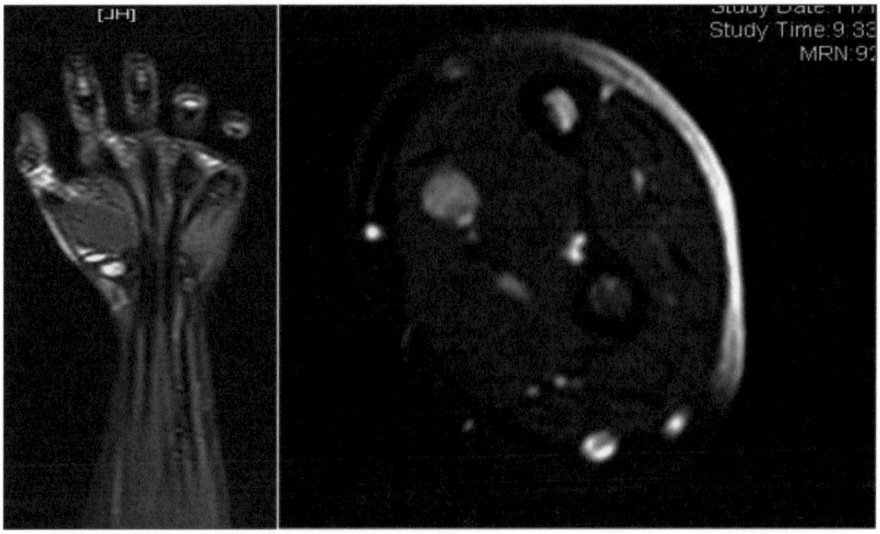

Figure 8.
Iatrogenic ulnar nerve lesion forearm segment with neuroma.

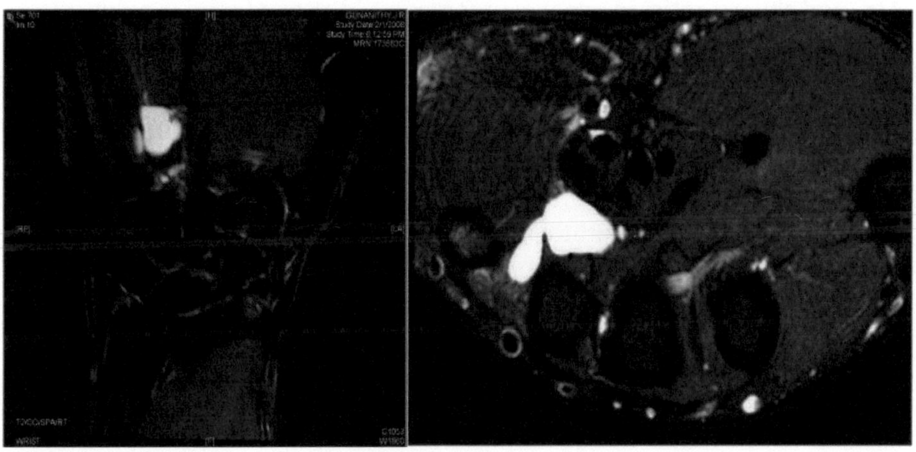

Figure 9.
Ganglion causing deep branch ulnar nerve compressive neuropathy.

15. Pitfalls in diagnosis

There could be errors in the diagnosis of neuropathies if one does not consider the clinical setting and if nerve conduction studies are not planned well and performed.

15.1 False positive

Lumbar canal stenosis with radiculopathy could sometimes be difficult to distinguish from polyneuropathy with distal sensory loss and absent ankle reflex. Intact

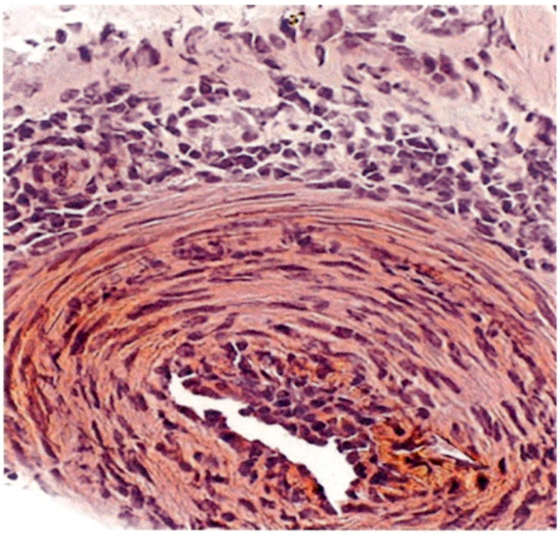

Figure 10.
Vasculitis showing inflammation around vessel wall with intact vessel wall. Vasculitis with peripheral neuropathy (non-systemic vasculitic neuropathy).

sensory nerve action potentials and denervation of proximal lower limb and paraspinal muscles in lumbar canal stenosis and low amplitude sensory nerve action potentials (SNAPs) and abnormalities in upper extremities could also be found in polyneuropathy.

Inclusion Myositis and distal spinal muscular atrophy could masquerade as a motor neuropathy.

In the elderly population, reduced vibration sense and absent ankle reflexes are not uncommon and nerve conduction studies could show low sural nerve sensory nerve action potentials, and one might overcall and need to interpret in the light of symptomatology.

Rarely, acute mononeuropathies involving radial, proximal median and peroneal nerve could mimic acute ischemic strokes, and careful attention to the weakness distribution would help in discerning.

Temperature-linked slowing of nerve conduction velocities can lead to erroneous diagnosis of CIDP and it's vital to warm the extremities.

There could be settings in which diagnosis of peripheral neuropathy is correct, but the cause is falsely attributed (see vignette 4-MNGIE).

15.2 False negative

False-negative diagnosis of peripheral neuropathy can occur in the setting of mild sensory polyneuropathy or small fiber neuropathy, with hardly any clinical findings when routine nerve conduction studies are normal.

16. Rating scales

Rating scales are required in research to better report outcome measures by standardizing the description of severity of disease and to monitor progression/response to treatment or interventions. Due to the heterogeneity of peripheral neuropathies, there is no designated gold standard scale yet for peripheral neuropathies.

List of scales used for studies in peripheral polyneuropathy over the years [28]:

- Clinical scales for peripheral neuropathy:
- Neurological Symptoms Scale
- Neuropathy Symptom Profile
- Neuropathy Disability Scale
- Overall Disability Sum Score (ODSS)
- Overall Neuropathy Limitation Scale (ONLS)
- Medical Research Council Sum Score
- Neuropathy Impairment Scale
- Inflammatory Neuropathy Cause and Treatment (INCAT) Sensory Sum Score
- Total Neuropathy Scale
- Veterans Affairs Neuropathy Scale
- Erasmus GBS Respiratory Insufficiency Score (EGRIS)

17. Treatment strategies

Treatment strategies include treating or removing the underlying cause and symptomatic management. The underlying etiology determines the type of treatment, and there have been evidence-based guidelines for treatment of Guillain-Barre syndrome and multifocal motor neuropathy. There is treatment algorithm for vasculitis-associated neuropathies, and it is always important to have pre-determined end points.

After evaluation, even after a specific etiology is found and targeted treatment is provided, the course of neuropathy can stabilize, and symptoms could improve but could be left with residual symptoms. Supportive and symptomatic care is paramount. The pain management includes anticonvulsant drugs, serotonin and noradrenaline reuptake inhibitors and tricyclic antidepressants. Patients who have lost sensations in their feet should be counseled on regular foot care and monitoring for wounds and injuries. Microvascular complications and diabetic neuropathy lead to the complication of diabetic foot, and the expenditure in the management of diabetic foot is quite high. Patients with muscle weakness would benefit from both physio- and occupational therapy and orthotics like ankle and foot and wrist and finger splints. Rehabilitation strategies are especially important in limiting disability and in preservation and maintenance of functional status.

18. Monitoring disease progression

Neuropathies need to be followed up to monitor the response to treatment modalities, both clinically and with follow up NCS/EMG. There is need to work closely with rehabilitation team including physio- and occupational therapy. Immune-mediated neuropathies especially require close follow up as they would need induction therapy followed by maintenance therapy. In the clinical setting, Medical Research Council (MRC) grading would be used to assess motor power, and in small fiber neuropathies, one might need protective foot gear and advice to avoid deformities.

19. Vignettes

Please find a few vignettes that would give an exposition to real-time scenarios:

19.1 Vignette 1: Acute inflammatory demyelinating polyradiculoneuropathy (AIDP)

A 26-year-old man presented to the emergency department with a 1-week history of ascending weakness with quadriparesis, preserved sensory and bladder/bowel function and was areflexic. He had an antecedent viral infection 3 weeks prior to the weakness. Nerve conduction studies show evidence of demyelinating polyradiculoneuropathy with proximal conduction block with sural sparing. CSF showed 2 lymphocytes with normal sugar and high protein. This is in keeping with a diagnosis of AIDP. He was treated with high dose IVIg 400 mg/kg/day x 5 days and received physiotherapy and occupational therapy. He responded to immunotherapy, and he made a good recovery in 8 weeks (**Table 6**).

19.2 Vignette 2: Critical illness neuropathy (CIN)

A 69-year-old man was admitted to the ICU for pneumonitis and sepsis and had to be ventilated for 2 weeks. There is significant PMHx of lung malignancy; he underwent lobectomy, chemo- and radiotherapy; and he has paroxysmal AF, for which he was on amiodarone. While in ICU, he was exposed to neuromuscular blocking agents (NMBA), corticosteroids, furosemide and colistin. The referral was for failure to wean off the ventilator. He was conscious, alert but had profound weakness of all 4 limbs with muscle wasting and areflexia. He was off NMBAs for over 48 h, and this

Motor Nerve Conduction:						
Nerve and Site	**Latency**	**Amplitude**	**Conduction Velocity**	**Duration**	**Latency Difference**	**Distance S**
Median.R						
Wrist	5.2 ms	12.3 mV	m/s	7.5 ms	ms	mm
Elbow	10.8 ms	10.3 mV	48 m/s	8.1 ms	5.6 ms	230 mm
Axilla	12.0 ms	9.5 mV	m/s	8.4 ms	1.2 ms	mm
Erbs points	17.3 ms	5.5 mV	m/s	10.6 ms	5.3 ms	mm
Median.L						
Wrist	6.5 ms	10.6 mV	m/s	8.8 ms	ms	mm
Elbow	12.0 ms	8.6 mV	49 m/s	9.2 ms	5.5 ms	230 mm
Axilla	13.2 ms	8.2 mV	m/s	9.3 ms	1.2 ms	mm
Erbs points	19.7 ms	4.9 mV	m/s	9.1 ms	6.5 ms	mm
Ulnar.R						

Motor Nerve Conduction:						
Nerve and Site	**Latency**	**Amplitude**	**Conduction Velocity**	**Duration**	**Latency Difference**	**Distance S**
Wrist	3.4 ms	10.7 mV	m/s	7.8 ms	ms	mm
Above elbow	11.7 ms	5.5 mV	37 m/s	8.1 ms	8.3 ms	310 mm
Below elbow	9.2 ms	8.0 mV	40 m/s	8.0 ms	2.5 ms	100 mm
Ulnar.L						
Wrist	3.3 ms	9.5 mV	m/s	8.5 ms	ms	mm
Above elbow	10.6 ms	8.1 mV	42 m/s	9.5 ms	7.3 ms	310 mm
Peroneal.R						
Ankle	5.4 ms	1.7 mV	m/s	9.3 ms	ms	mm
Fibula (head)	17.2 ms	0.9 mV	36 m/s	8.2 ms	11.8 ms	420 mm
Peroneal.L						
Ankle	6.2 ms	4.9 mV	m/s	7.9 ms	ms	mm
Fibula (head)	17.3 ms	3.2 mV	38 m/s	8.8 ms	11.1 ms	420 mm
Tibial.R						
Ankle	6.7 ms	2.0 mV	m/s	11.6 ms	ms	mm
Popliteal fossa	18.9 ms	1.2 mV	36 m/s	11.9 ms	12.2 ms	440 mm
Tibial.L						
Ankle	7.5 ms	2.3 mV	m/s	10.6 ms	ms	mm
Popliteal fossa	21.0 ms	1.0 mV	33 m/s	13.0 ms	13.5 ms	440 mm
Recording on TAL						
Right	5.5 ms	4.0 mV	m/s	ms	5.5 ms	mm
Left	5.3 ms	4.2 mV	m/s	15.4 ms	0.2 ms	mm
Facial.L						
RIGHT	5.2 ms	3.3 mV	m/s	8.6 ms	0.5 ms	mm
Facial.R						
LEFT	4.7 ms	3.2 mV	m/s	7.6 ms	ms	mm
Phrenic.R						
Right	11.3 ms	0.3 mV	m/s	ms	11.3 ms	mm
Left	10.4 ms	0.3 mV	m/s	ms	10.4 ms	mm

F-Wave Studies	
Nerve	**F-Latency**
Median.R	30.2 ms
Median.L	34.7 ms
Ulnar.R	31.1 ms
Ulnar.L	34.8 ms
Peroneal.R	64.5 ms
Peroneal.L	64.8 ms

F-Wave Studies	
Nerve	**F-Latency**
Tibial.R	73.8 ms
Tibial.L	76.2 ms

H-waves:		
Nerve	**Latency**	**Amplitude (max)**
Tibial.R		
H-wave:	Not Obtained	
Tibial.L		
H-wave:	Not Obtained	

Sensory Nerve Conduction:						
Nerve and Site	**Distal Latency**	**Amplitude**	**Conduction Velocity**	**Segment**	**Latency Difference**	**Distance S**
Median.R						
Wrist	2.2 ms	6 μV	51 m/s	Digit II (index finger)-Wrist	2.2 ms	110 mm
Median.L						
Wrist	3.4 ms	6 μV	35 m/s	Digit II (index finger)-Wrist	3.4 ms	120 mm
Ulnar.R						
Wrist	2.0 ms	14 μV	54 m/s	Digit V (little finger)-Wrist	2.0 ms	110 mm
Ulnar.L						
Wrist	2.7 ms	8 μV	43 m/s	Digit V (little finger)-Wrist	2.7 ms	115 mm
Sural.R						
Lower leg	1.9 ms	22 μV	59 m/s	Ankle-Lower leg	1.9 ms	110 mm
Sural.L						
Lower leg	1.7 ms	27 μV	65 m/s	Ankle-Lower leg	1.7 ms	110 mm
Superficial peroneal.R						
Ankle	2.4 ms	16 μV	42 m/s	Dorsum of foot-Ankle	2.4 ms	100 mm
Superficial peroneal.L						
Ankle	2.4 ms	22 μV	42 m/s	Doesum of foot-Ankle	2.4 ms	100 mm

Table 6.
Nerve conduction studies of the patient with AIDP.

was the setting for critical illness neuropathy (CIN). NCS shows severe reduction of motor CMAPs of upper and lower limbs, and sensory nerve action potentials were reduced. The phrenic nerves were inexcitable and received physiotherapy but had a prolonged ICU stay and succumbed to severe sepsis after 10 weeks. CIN is an important cause of ICU-acquired paresis and is important to recognize as this has implications for problems in weaning off the ventilator and resultant prolonged ICU stay.

19.3 Vignette 3: Diabetes with lumbosacral radiculoplexopathy

A 77-year-old man with PMHx of diabetes mellitus presented with 2 months history of intermediate-proximal weakness of the right lower limb, which then progressed to the distal group and then spread to the left lower limb. O/E The motor power was grade 2/5 in right lower limb, proximo-intermediate and distal group of muscles and left lower limb was grade 3–4/5 weakness of proximal group and 4/5 in intermediate-distal group in the left lower limb. Sensory impairment distal to ankle and also in lateral cutaneous nerve of thigh distribution on right side and deep tendon reflexes were absent. Nerve conduction studies showed evidence of lumbosacral radiculoplexopathy. MRI of the lumbosacral spine showed enhancement of lumbosacral plexus. The right superficial fibular nerve biopsy shows evidence of asymmetrical nerve fibers with Wallerian degeneration. He was treated with pulse IV cyclophosphamide, pulse IV methylprednisolone and physiotherapy and made a very good recovery with improvement in motor power of lower limbs, and in a years' time, he was ambulant without walking aid (**Figure 11**).

19.4 Vignette 4: MNGIE

A 21-year-old man presented with recurrent episodes of weakness of all 4 limbs, precipitated by fever with autonomic disturbances and failure to thrive. There is a family history of his sister being affected and was being treated as a CIDP but succumbed to illness. NCS showed demyelinating neuropathy, CPK was 4680 IU, and blood lactate was 2. MRI brain showed diffuse white matter hyperintensity. Autonomic function testing showed GI dysmotility and orthostatic hypotension. Biochemical screening showed thymidine phosphorylase deficiency (< 10% of normal assay). The diagnosis was mitochondrial neurogastrointestinal encephalopathy (MNGIE), and he was treated with hemodialysis followed by peritoneal dialysis. He had a protracted recovery and autonomic symptoms abated and neuropathy improved with weight gain (**Figure 12**).

19.5 Vignette 5: Sciatic neuropathy

A 65-year-old man presented with a 10 days history of gluteal pain, tingling of dorsal surface of foot followed by weakness of dorsiflexors, plantar flexors, evertors and invertors of right foot, and there was a history of an invasive procedure to the right hip 2 weeks ago. Nerve conductions showed evidence of a right sciatic neuropathy, with fibular more involved than tibial nerve. MRI of pelvis showed a hypointense lesion in piriformis fossa, which was evaluated with CT pelvis and CT angiogram done to rule out a pseudoaneurysm that showed a hematoma at the greater sciatic foramen causing compression of the right sciatic nerve (**Figure 13**).

The hematoma was evacuated by the surgeons, and the patient improved with physiotherapy but had residual foot drop requiring orthosis for a period of 1 year.

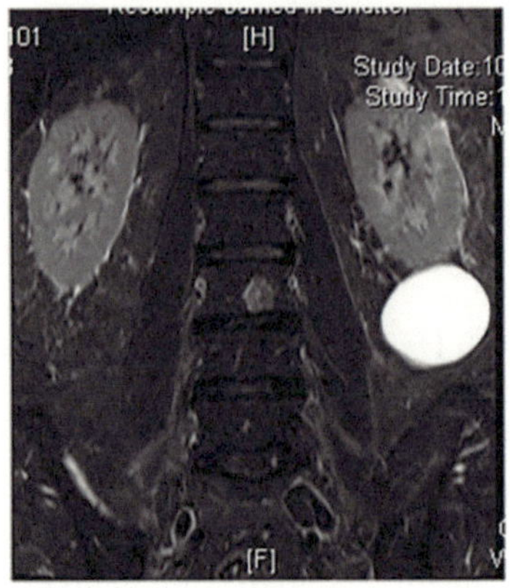

Figure 11.
MRI showing right lumbosacral plexus thickening with mild hyperintensity.

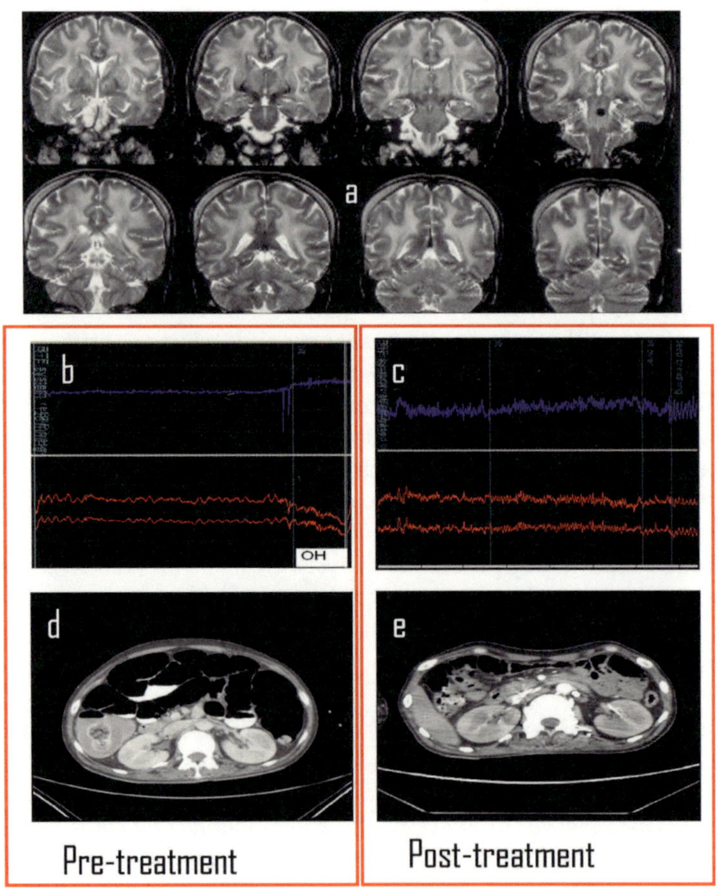

a: Features of Leukoencephalopathy.
b: beat to beat record with OH. c: Resolution of OH after Rx.
c: dilated loops of intestine. d: normal loops of intestine after Rx

Figure 12.
MRI brain, Autonomic Function Tests and CT abdomen in the pt with MNGIE – Sivadasan and Alexander [29].

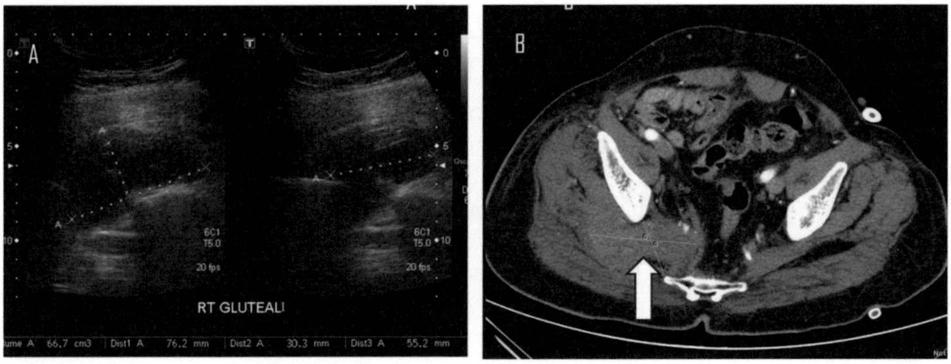

Figure 13.
(A. Ultrasound; B: CT Pelvis): Hematoma in the right greater sciatic foramen with compression of sciatic nerve.

19.6 Vignette 6: Post-infectious pan-dysautonomia

A 30-year-old lady was admitted with a 2-month history of abdominal pain, vomiting, diarrhea, postural giddiness and syncope. There is an antecedent illness of mumps 2 weeks before the illness. There is no motor weakness and cranial neuropathy, and deep tendon reflexes were elicited. Bed side autonomic tests were abnormal including cold pressor test, Valsalva, E-I ratio, supine to standing heart rate response were all abnormal. Workup for porphyria and toxins was negative and CSF was acellular with protein of 70 mg and sugar was normal. Mumps antibody was negative. She was treated with IVIg and fludrocortisone. There was improvement, both clinically and on AFT, and by 1 month, she was normal with normal AFT.

Serial Bedside Autonomic Function Testing (**Table 7**).

Parameter **Date**	**21/07/1997**	**03/08/1997**	**02/09/1997**
Supine BP, systolic/diastolic (mm Hg)	130/90	140/90	116/82
Erect BP, systolic/ diastolic (mm Hg)*	90/70	110/70	110/80
Supine pulse rate (beats/min)	94	92	86
Erect pulse rate (beats/min)**	110	108	102
Cold pressor test- Baseline BP (mm Hg)	128/90	130/90	110/80
Cold pressor test- BP with 5 min immersion (mm Hg) †	128/90	140/90	120/86
Isometric exercise - Baseline BP (mmHg)	130/80	130/90	110/80
Isometric exercise - BP with 5 min sustained hand grip ‡	130/100	130/80	120/80
Expiration to inspiration ratio on ECG ∫	1.12	1.18	1.21
Valsalva maneuver- longest R-R / shortest R-R on ECG ∮	1.13	1.38	1.43
RR ratio- 30th beat to 15th beat after standing on ECG ∯	0.86	0.93	1.07

**Normal fall in systolic/diastolic BP < 30/15 mmHg on standing.*
***Normal increase in pulse rate of 11–29 beats/min on standing.*
† Normal increase in BP by 15-20 mm Hg systolic or 10–15 mm Hg diastolic.
‡ Normal increase in diastolic BP by 15 mm Hg.
∫ Normal >1.2.
∮ Normal >1.4.
∯ Normal >1.04.
RR – distance between 2 successive R waves on ECG in seconds.
Ref. [30].

Table 7.
Bed side autonomic function testing in pt with acute Pan-dysautonomia.

19.7 Vignette 7: Neurolymphomatosis (primary)

A 67-year-old man presented with a 2-week history of pain and weakness in the left arm and forearm. On examination, there was swelling of the left supraclavicular region. MRI of cervical spine including brachial plexus showed an elongated mass along the left C7 nerve and extending into the brachial plexus. Ultrasound showed a lamellated appearance of the mass with preserved nerve architecture. He also had a recent onset of significant loss of weight and change in bowel habits. Whole-body PET CT showed high standardized uptake value (SUV) lesion in the left brachial plexus, right lumbar and lumbosacral plexus, and presacral plexus. There was a swelling in the left L3 nerve extending into paraspinal muscle, which was biopsied, and

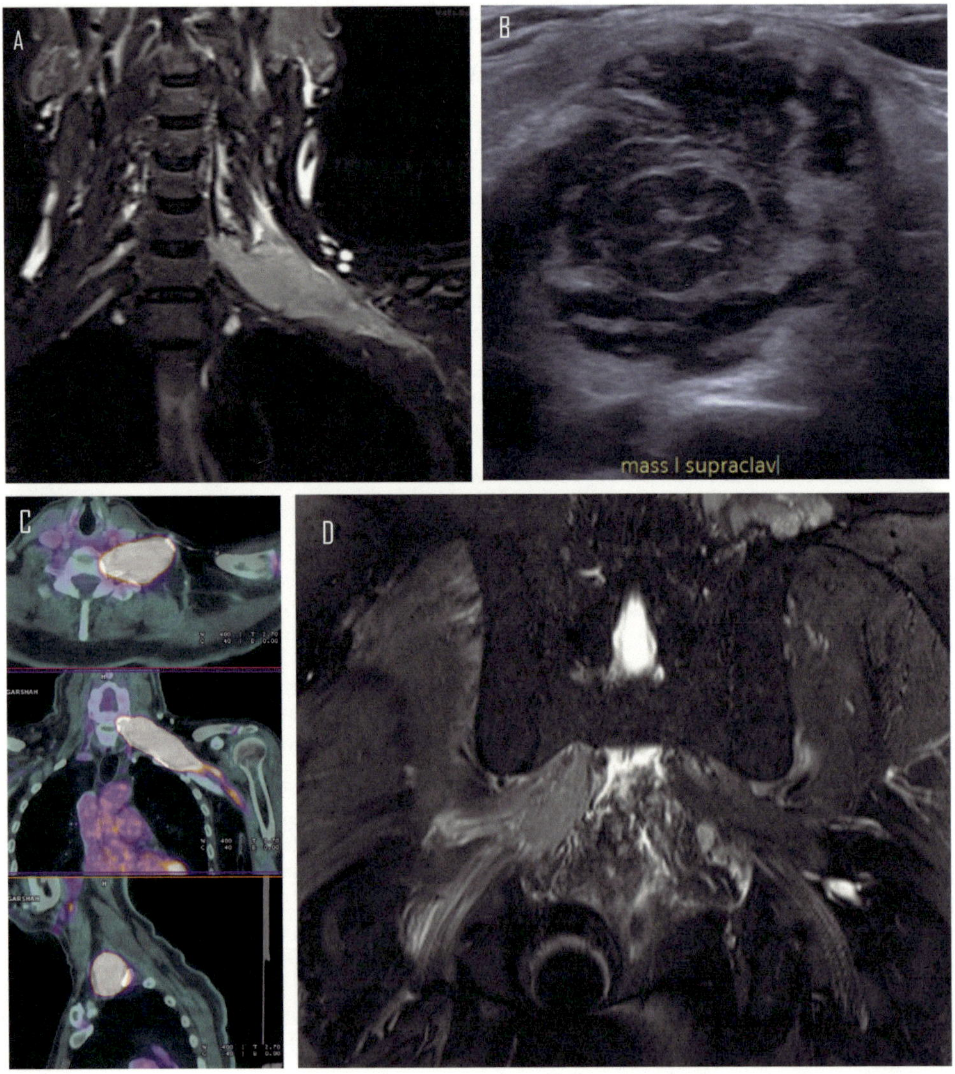

Figure 14.
A. MRI shows an elongated soft tissue mass involving left brachial plexus; B. US showing expanded brachial plexus with preserved architecture; C. PET CT showing high SUV uptake from left brachial plexus; D. MRI showing enlargement of right lumbosacral plexus.

the tissue diagnosis showed diffuse large B cell lymphoma (neurolymphomatosis). The presence of severe pain, where one needs to try anticonvulsant drugs, SNRI and tricyclic antidepressant drugs, should alert the clinician that the nature of brachial plexopathy to be an infiltrative pathology and investigate appropriately. He was started on R-EPOCH regime by the oncologist, and a repeat MR imaging of brachial plexus 8 weeks after chemotherapy showed significant reduction in size of the brachial plexus mass lesion, which corroborated with clinical improvement (**Figure 14**).

20. Conclusion

This chapter has attempted to give a comprehensive overview on the approach to peripheral neuropathy and hope this could be a good reference, when one encounters this disorder. The field of polyneuropathies is quite vast, and authors would recommend more focused reading on the etiopathogenesis, electrophysiology, pathology, evidence-based treatment guidelines, rehabilitation strategies and outcome.

Acknowledgements

The authors would like to express their heartfelt gratitude to Dr. Madhavi K, Professor of Radiodiagnosis, Christian Medical College and Hospital, Vellore, India, and Dr. Sunithi Elizabeth Mani, Consultant Radiologist, Jerudong Park Medical Centre, Brunei, for contributing the radiological images for the manuscript and to all our patients over the years who have enriched our repertoire.

Author details

Chee Shin Yong[1] and Mathew Alexander[2]*

1 Neurology Department, Brunei Neuroscience Stroke and Rehabilitation Centre, PJSC, Brunei Darussalam

2 Department of Neurological Sciences, Christian Medical College and Hospital, Vellore, India

*Address all correspondence to: mathewalex59@gmail.com

References

[1] Martyn CN, Hughes RA. Epidemiology of peripheral neuropathy. Journal of Neurology, Neurosurgery, and Psychiatry. 1997;**62**(4):310-318. DOI: 10.1136/jnnp.62.4.310

[2] Trivedi S, Pandit A, Ganguly G, Das SK. Epidemiology of peripheral neurology: An Indian perspective. Annals of Indian Academy of Neurology. 2017;**20**(3):173-184. DOI: 10.4103/aian.AIAN_470_16

[3] England JD, Asbury AK. Peripheral neuropathy. Lancet. 2004;**363**(9427):2151-2161. DOI: 10.1016/S0140-6736(04) 16508-2

[4] Farhad K, Traub R, Ruzhansky KM, Brannagan TH 3rd. Causes of neuropathy in patients referred as "idiopathic neuropathy". Muscle and Nerve. 2016;**53**(6):856-861. DOI: 1.1002/mus.24969

[5] Barohn RJ, Amato AA. Pattern-recognition approach to neuropathy and neuronopathy. Neurologic Clinics. 2013;**31**(2):343-361. DOI: 10.101/j.ncl.2013.02.001

[6] Asbury AK, Gilliat RW. Peripheral Nerve Disorders - A Practical Approach. Oxford, UK: Butterworths; 1984. ISBN:978-0407022973/040670229X

[7] Vinik A, Ullal J, Parson HK, Casellini CM. Diabetic neuropathies: Clinical manifestations and current treatment options. Nature Clinical Practice Endocrinology and Metabolism. 2006;**2**(5):269-281. DOI: 10.1038/ncpendmet0142

[8] Erlanger J, Gasser HS. Electrical Signs of Nervous Activity. Philadelphia: University of Pennsylvania Press; 1968. ISBN 09780812275865/0812275861

[9] Whitwam JG. Classification of peripheral nerve fibres. An Historical Perspective. Anaesthesia. 1976;**31**(4):494-503. DOI: 10.111/j.1365-2044.1976.tb12354.x

[10] Herrmann DN, Griffin JW, Hauer P, Cornblath DR, McArthur JC. Epidermal nerve fiber density and sural nerve morphometry in peripheral neuropathies. Neurology. 1999;**53**(8):1634-1640. DOI: 10.1212/wnl.53.8.1634

[11] Periquet MI, Novak V, Collins MP, Nagaraj HN, Erdem S, Nash SM, et al. Painful sensory neuropathy: Prospective evaluation using skin biopsy. Neurology. 1999;**53**(8):1641-1647. DOI: 10.1212/wnl.53.8.1641

[12] Herrmann DN, Logigian EL. Approach to Peripheral Nerve Disorders in Neuromuscular Disorders in Clinical Practice-Second Edition. New York City, New York: Springer; 2013. pp. 495-505

[13] Katriji B, Ruff R. Kaminski HJ Neuromuscular Disorders in Clinical Practice. 2nd ed. New York City, New York: Springer; 2013. ISBN 9781493942374/1493942379

[14] Watson JC, Dyck PJB. Peripheral neuropathy: A practical approach to diagnosis and symptom management. Mayo Clinic Proceedings. 2015;**9**(7):940-951. DOI: 10.1016/j.mayocp.2015.05.004

[15] Smyth D, Kramarz C, Carr AS, Rossor AM, Lunn MP. Toxic neuropathies: A practical approach. Practical Neurology. 2023;**23**(2):120-130. DOI: 10.1136/on-2022-003444

[16] England JD, Gronseth GS, Franklin G. Practice parameter: Evaluation of distal symmetric polyneuropathy: Role of autonomic testing, nerve biopsy, and skin biopsy (an evidence-based review). Report of the American Academy of Neurology, American Association of Neuromuscular and Electrodiagnostic Medicine, and American Academy of physical medicine and rehabilitation. Neurology. 2009;**72**(2):177-184. DOI: 10.1212/01.wnl.0000336345.0f

[17] Sapporta AS, Sottile SL, Millie LJ, Feely SM, Siskind CE, Sy ME. Charcot–Marie-tooth disease subtypes and genetic testing strategies. Annals of Neurology. 2011;**69**(1):22-33. DOI: 10.1002/ana.22166

[18] Griffin JW, Hseih ST, McArthur JC, Cornblath DR. Laboratory testing in peripheral neuropathies. Neurologic Clinics. 1996;**14**(1):119-133. DOI: 10.1016/s0733-8610(05)70246-2

[19] Kieseier BC, Mathew E, Sommer C, Hartung HP. Immune-mediated neuropathies. Nature Reviews Disease Primers. 2018;**4**(1):31. DOI: 10.1038/s41572-018-0027-2

[20] Wolfe GI, El-Feky WH, Katz JS, Bryan WW, Wians FH Jr, Barohn RJ. Antibody panels in idiopathic polyneuropathy and motor neuron diseases. Muscle and Nerve. 1997;**20**(10):1275-1283. DOI: 10.1002/(sici)1097-4598(199710)2-:10>1275::AID-MUS10>3.0;2-2

[21] Rossor AM, Reilly MM. Blood biomarkers of peripheral neuropathy. Acta Neurologica Scandinavica. 2022;**146**(4):325-331. DOI: 10.1111/ane.13650

[22] Rossor AM, Evans MR, Reilly MM. A practical approach to the genetic neuropathies. Practical Neurology. 2015;**15**(3):187-198. DOI: 10.1136/practneurol-2015-001095

[23] Yablon CM, Hammer MR, Morag Y, Brandon CJ, Fessell DP, Jacobson JA. US of the peripheral nerves of the lower extremity: A landmark approach. Radiographics. 2016;**36**(2):468-474. DOI: 10.1148/rg.2016150120

[24] Zaidman CM, Seelig MJ, Baker JC, Mackinnon SE, Pestronk A. Detection of peripheral nerve pathology: Comparison of ultrasound and MRI. Neurology. 2013;**80**(18):1634-1640. DOI: 10.1212/WNL.0b013e3182904f3f

[25] Soldatos T, Andreisek G, Thawait GK, Guggenberger R, Williams EH, Carrino JA, et al. High resolution 3-T MR neurography of the lumbosacral plexus. Radiographics. 2013;**33**(4):967-987. DOI: 10.1148/rg.334115761

[26] Sureka J, Cherian RA, Alexander M, Thomas BP. MRI of brachial plexopathies. Clinical Radiology. 2009;**64**(2):208-218. DOI: 10.1016/j.crad.2008.08.011

[27] Nathani D, Spies J, Barnett MH, Pollar J, Wang MX, Sommer C, et al. Nerve biopsy: Current indications and decision tools. Muscle and Nerve. 2021;**64**(2):125-139. DOI: 10/1002/mus.27201

[28] Hanewinckel R, Ikram MA, Van Doorn PA. Assessment scales for the diagnosis of polyneuropathy. Journal of the Peripheral Nervous System. 2016;**21**(2):61-73. DOI: 19.1111/jns.12170

[29] Sivadasan A, Muthusamy K, Patil AK, Mathew V, Alexander M. Pearls and Oy-sters: Mitochondrial neurogastrointestinal

encephalomyelopathy diagnosis and response to peritoneal dialysis. Neurology. 2016;**86**(14):e147-e150. DOI: 10.1212/WNL.0000000000002536

[30] Venkatraman S, Alexander M, Gnanamuthu C. Postinfectious pandysautonomia with complete recovery after intravenous immunoglobulin therapy. Neurology. 1998;**51**(6):1764-1765. DOI: 10.1212/wnl.51.6.1764

Chapter 5

More Consumption of Ultra-Processed and Sugar-Sweetened Beverages Could Increase Odds of Sarcopenia in Kidney Diseases

Marzieh Mahmoodi, Fatemeh Mansouri, Maede Makhtoomi, Zainab Shateri and Mehran Nouri

Abstract

Chronic kidney disease (CKD) is a degenerative condition characterized by the gradual deterioration of renal function. Among the risk factors for the disease, older age, ethnicity, low birth weight, and family history of kidney disease are the most important. Other significant risk factors include smoking, obesity, hypertension, uncontrolled diabetes mellitus, exposure to heavy metals, chronic alcohol consumption, and the use of analgesic medications. Findings have also shown the relationship between CKD and sarcopenia. The prevalence of sarcopenia increases with the severity of CKD, independent of the definition of sarcopenia used. Muscle wasting in CKD is multifactorial. Several factors related to the development of chronic kidney failure lead to muscle loss, making CKD an independent risk factor for sarcopenia. Increasing age and female gender are known as non-modifiable risk factors for sarcopenia, while dietary intake is considered a modifiable risk factor. In the elderly, nutritional imbalances have been reported due to age-related physiological changes, such as loss of appetite, diminished senses of taste and thirst, and impaired nutrient absorption and utilization. Poor diet quality can potential increase the risk of worsening sarcopenia in CKD patients. Therefore, nutritional recommendations for CKD patients should emphasize nutrient-dense foods to support overall health and mitigate the risk of sarcopenia.

Keywords: kidney diseases, sarcopenia, sugar-sweetened beverages, ultra-processed food, diet, nutritional intake

1. Introduction

Chronic kidney disease (CKD) is a degenerative condition characterized by the gradual deterioration of renal function. Its affects about 10% of the world's population [1].

IntechOpen

Reported findings indicate an increasing trend in the prevalence of the disease worldwide [2]. The results obtained from a systematic analysis of population-based data worldwide have demonstrated that the age-standardized global prevalence of CKD stages 1–5 in among individuals aged 20 years and older in men and women is 10.4 and 11.8%, respectively [3]. In another study, geographical differences based on income level were found to significantly influence CKD prevalence [2]. Age-standardized CKD prevalence rates in high-income countries are 8.6% in men and 9.6% in women, while in medium and low-income countries, rates are reported as 10.6% in men and 12.5% in women [2].

In addition, the age-standardized global prevalence of CKD stages 3–5 in adults aged 20 years and older is reported as 4.7% in men and 5.8% in women [2]. In a recent systematic review and meta-analysis study that examined 6,908,404 patients across 100 studies, the global prevalence of CKD stages 1–5 was reported as 13.4%. For CKD stages 3–5, the prevalence was 10.6%. These finding provide valuable insights into the global burden of CKD [4]. Moreover, according to the findings, the total number of people worldwide with CKD stages 1–5 is approximately 843.6 million [2].

2. Risk factors

Chronic kidney disease has become a significant public health issue. Therefore, early intervention is crucial to mitigate its economic burden. This necessitates through investigation and identification of the diseases risk factors [5]. Among the risk factors of the disease, older age, African American descent, low birth weight, and family history of kidney disease are the most important factors [5]. Additionally, smoking, obesity, hypertension, uncontrolled diabetes mellitus, exposure to heavy metals, chronic alcohol consumption, and the use of analgesic medications are also significant risk factors [5].

Research demonstrates a relationship between CKD and sarcopenia, where the prevalence of sarcopenia increases with the severity of CKD regardless of its definition [6]. To understand the pathophysiology of sarcopenia in CKD, it is crucial to recognize that muscle wasting in CKD is multifactorial [6]. Several factors associated with the progression of chronic kidney failure contribute to muscle loss, establishing CKD as an independent risk factor for sarcopenia [6]. Sarcopenia and CKD are both progressive diseases sharing similar pathophysiological pathways and risk factors [6].

Muscle homeostasis relies on balancing anabolism and catabolism. In CKD, muscle loss occurs due to increased catabolism, involving activation of pathways like the ubiquitin-proteasome system, caspase 3, and lysosomes. Additionally, CKD impairs muscle growth, regeneration, and protein synthesis [6].

The decline in myogenesis is attributed to impaired function of muscle precursor (satellite) cells in individuals with CKD [6]. Several factors contribute to this imbalance in individuals with CKD, including metabolic acidosis, endocrine disorders affecting insulin-IGF-1 signaling, low testosterone levels, alterations in the renin-angiotensin-aldosterone system, systemic inflammation, and dysregulation of hypothalamic appetite control [6].

3. Definition of sarcopenia

Sarcopenia is a progressive disorder characterized by decreased muscle strength (dynapenia), reduced muscle mass, and impaired muscle function [7]. For the first time in 1989, Rosenberg defined sarcopenia as an age-related decrease in muscle mass in his publication [8]. Recently, the European Working Groups on Sarcopenia in Older People (EWGSOP), the European Society for Clinical Nutrition and Metabolism Special Interest Groups (ESPEN-SIG), and the International Working Group on Sarcopenia (IWGS) have defined sarcopenia, each providing distinct criteria and perspectives [8].

According to the EWGSOP, sarcopenia is defined as a decrease in muscle mass accompanied by a decrease in muscle strength or function. ESPEN-SIG considers sarcopenia as the loss of muscle mass and strength. IWGS defines sarcopenia as decreased muscle mass and decreased muscle function, which may be associated with either decreased muscle mass alone or increased fat mass. According to the definition of EWGSOP, severe sarcopenia is characterized by decreases in all three aspects: muscle mass, strength, and function [8–10].

AWGS, like other groups, defines sarcopenia as a reduction in muscle mass, strength, or performance [8]. In general, sarcopenia is recognized as a progressive musculoskeletal syndrome associated with age-related declines in muscle mass, strength, and function [11]. Sarcopenia plays an important role in physiological and cognitive decline and is associated with an increased risk of death, disability, falls, and hospitalization [7, 12]. A gradual decrease in muscle mass and strength due to muscle atrophy and cell death has been reported in individuals starting from the sixth decade of life [12].

4. Prevalence of sarcopenia

A 30% decrease in muscle mass has been reported in 80-year-old adults, with greater changes observed in fiber size and number, particularly affecting type 2 fibers [12, 13]. A decline in muscle strength also has been shown with age [14]. Sarcopenia is a common condition in elderly individuals over 65 years old, with reported prevalence rates ranging between 10% and 50% depending on varying definitions and study populations [15].

5. Risk factors for sarcopenia

Neurological factors associated with the lack of motor neurons, endocrine changes due to the reduced of hormone expressions such as growth hormone (GH) and testosterone, loss of muscle motor units, and lifestyle and nutritional changes related to the adaptation of sedentary habits are all recognized as contributing causes of sarcopenia [12]. Therefore, sarcopenia is often observed during periods of life characterized by significantly reduced physical activity, as documented in various studies on aging and muscle health [12, 16]. Age, sex, low physical activity, poor diet, and chronic inflammation are recognized as risk factors for sarcopenia, a multifactorial disease affecting muscle health [15].

6. Effect of hormones on the progression of sarcopenia in CKD

Hormones play an important role in the development of sarcopenia by affecting muscle mass and muscle strength in patients with CKD. These hormones include testosterone, growth hormone, insulin, thyroid hormones, and vitamin D [17].

6.1 Testosterone

A high risk of muscular atrophy and sarcopenia in CKD patients has been reported due to testosterone deficiency, CKD-related complications, inflammation, and malnutrition (hormones) [17]. Testosterone is an anabolic hormone required for protein synthesis, muscle mass, and muscle strength, leading to increased protein synthesis and decreased protein catabolism [17]. Therefore, the decrease in testosterone levels in CKD patients leads to an increase in myostatin expression as a hormone secreted by the muscle, which prevents muscle growth and damage to IGF-1 signal transduction [17]. In addition, testosterone deficiency leads to an increase in the level of the pro-inflammatory cytokine, disruption in mesenchymal stem cell differentiation, increase in adipocyte progenitor cells and fat storage in muscles, and mitochondrial degradation [17]. Therefore, testosterone deficiency is involved in the development of sarcopenia through the mentioned mechanisms [17].

6.2 Vitamin D

Vitamin D is an important molecule of muscle and bone physiology, which regulates myokines and osteokines of muscle and bone such as vascular endothelial 1, growth factor, insulin-like growth factor 1, follistatin, fibroblast growth factor, osteoglycin, sclerostin, and osteocalcin [17]. One of the reasons that CKD patients are prone to sarcopenia is vitamin D deficiency [17]. An increase in FGF-23, decrease in kidney mass, dietary restriction, nutritional deficiencies, decrease in vitamin D receptor, reabsorption damage due to megalin in the proximal tubule, decrease in skin synthesis of vitamin D, and accumulation of uremic and proteinuria toxins are the factors that cause vitamin D deficiency in kidney patients [17]. This deficiency is effective in causing sarcopenia by decreasing type 2 muscle fibers, increasing the expression of myostatin, and decreasing the level of sclerostin and follistatin, and IGF-1, FGF, and VEGF [17].

6.3 Growth hormone

Because of the kidney's role in the elimination of growth hormone, the half-life of growth hormone is prolonged in CKD patients [17]. Metabolic acidosis, inflammation, reduced food intake, and uremia play a role in reducing the effectiveness of growth hormones [17]. Various factors play a role in growth hormone resistance in CKD patients, including suppression of cytokine signaling, changes in the GH/IGF-1 axis, reduction of hepatic receptor mRNA, IGF-1 inhibitors, and reduction of serum GHBP concentration and activity [17]. The GH/IGF-1 axis plays a key role in the pathogenesis of sarcopenia in CKD patients by causing inflammation [17]. Therefore, due to the anti-inflammatory properties of GH-based therapies, it is suggested to conduct more studies to use them to manage sarcopenia in patients with CKD [17].

6.4 Thyroid hormone

It has been shown that low levels of thyroid hormone T_3 and subclinical hypothyroidism due to decreased iodine clearance and chronic inflammation are common in patients with CKD [17]. Although skeletal muscles are one of the main target tissues of thyroid hormone and these hormones affect muscle growth, contraction/relaxation cycle, energy provision, and glucose homeostasis in muscles, there is no still clear and comprehensive evidence of the effect of thyroid hormones on sarcopenia in CKD patients [17]. Therefore, it is important to check the level of thyroid hormones in this category of patients and, if necessary, replace them with positive effects [17].

6.5 Insulin resistance

Insulin resistance has been reported in patients with CKD and is often associated with disease progression [17]. Chronic inflammation, oxidative stress, vitamin D deficiency, metabolic acidosis, anemia, and unknown uremic toxins are known possible causes of insulin resistance. Although the main reasons for CKD are unknown [17]. The relationship between insulin resistance and sarcopenia may be a description of the sarcopenic obesity condition, which is characterized by the accumulation of fat in the skeletal muscles [17]. Although a new therapeutic agent for insulin resistance in patients with CKD has not been reported, insulin resistance and sarcopenia may be considered as a new target for further studies [17].

7. Nutrition and sarcopenia

Increasing age and female gender are widely recognized as non-modifiable risk factors for sarcopenia, while dietary intake is acknowledged as a modifiable risk factor, as considered in recent reviews on sarcopenia [8]. In the elderly, nutritional imbalances have been reported due to age-related physiological changes, including documented loss of appetite, sensory perception affecting taste and thirst, and reduced nutrient absorption and utilization [18]. Decreased protein intake is considered a serious problem among the elderly due to documented issues such as poor appetite, chewing problems, and associated mental, social, and financial challenges [18]. This decrease in protein intake and increase in protein requirement during this period has been documented to disturb the balance between protein synthesis and breakdown, ultimately leading to skeletal muscle mass loss [18]. Because poor diet and nutritional status are common in the elderly, especially vulnerable individuals, sarcopenia has been reported to be associated with nutrient deficiencies stemming from low dietary intake in this population [8]. Therefore, the role of nutrition in preventing and treating sarcopenia is very important [8, 19]. It has been shown that food quantity, quality, and energy consumption play significant roles as risk factors for sarcopenia [20].

Loss of muscle mass is a common complication in patients with chronic kidney disease, the etiology of which is multifactorial and may be due to typical low-grade inflammation conditions in chronic kidney patients, insulin resistance, metabolic acidosis, vitamin D deficiency, imbalance in hormonal level, amino acid loss during dialysis, and decrease in dietary intake [21]. All these conditions are involved in increasing protein degradation and decreasing protein synthesis, thus creating a negative protein balance [21]. Therefore, appropriate nutrition and diet recommendations are important in preventing nutritional deficiencies and muscle wasting in CKD patients [21]. In this regard, low protein diets (LPDs) and very low protein diets (VLPDs) supplemented with amino acids or keto acids are common because of the role of protein restriction in managing uremic toxins and slowing the progression of CKD [21]. However, the relationship between excessive protein restriction and muscle weakness should be noted, and this is a controversial issue because protein restriction is effective in reducing the risk of worsening kidney function, but it may increase the risk of sarcopenia [22]. On the other hand, despite the contradictory findings related to the lack of essential amino acids following adhering to plant-based diets, evidence has shown that balanced and diverse plant-based diets are nutritionally sufficient [22]. In this regard, it has been shown that adherence to a Mediterranean dietary pattern rich in fruits and vegetables, legumes, and cereals may reduce the progression of CKD and related complications [22]. The protective effects of a vegetable-based diet on muscle strength have not been comprehensively explained [22]. Still, this hypothesis has been proposed according to the findings that alkaline diets, such as those rich in vegetables, play a role in maintaining muscle mass by reducing metabolic acidosis. However, the exact mechanism of the effect of a vegetable-based diet on muscle mass and counter with sarcopenia needs more research [22].

8. Sugar-sweetened beverages (SSB) and sarcopenia

Adequate fluid intake in the elderly has been shown to improve physical and mental performance, reducing the risk of falls, constipation, confusion, and cognitive impairment [23]. Beverages, such as water and juices, play a vital role in maintaining hydraulic balance, with some containing essential nutrients and bioactive components that contribute to overall health status [24]. In the US diet, added sugar is a significant component, contributing an average of 13.6% to the energy intake of the elderly's diet, as reported by recent dietary surveys [25]. The World Health Organization (WHO) and the 2015 Dietary Guidelines Advisory Committee (DGAC) recommend a maximum of 10% of energy intake from sugar. However, a study indicates that 65% of the elderly consume more than this recommended amount [25].

Added sugar in the liquid source form of the American diet primarily comes from SSBs (37.1 percent) and fruit drinks (8.9 percent) [25]. This dietary pattern can lead to increased energy intake and substitution of nutrient-rich diet components, potentially increasing the risk of malnutrition in the elderly [25]. Therefore, SSBs are recognized as a significant source of added sugar in the diet, rich in refined carbohydrates [26]. Their consumption is notably increasing in developing countries, contributing to dietary trends [27]. A positive association of SSB consumption and increased risk of chronic disorders has been documented in several studies [27–29].

The results obtained from the cohort study by Heo et al. have shown that consuming more than one serving of sugar-sweetened beverages or any amount of artificially sweetened beverages has led to an increased risk of CKD [30]. Similarly, in 1690 participants in the Tehran Glucose and Lipid Study without CKD, it has also been shown that the consumption of sugar-sweetened beverages is associated with an increased risk of CKD [31]. Sugar-sweetened beverages are known as an important source of free sugars, which due to high glycemic load is associated with metabolic changes related to diabetes such as increased blood glucose and hyperinsulinemia, resulting in impaired glucose tolerance and insulin resistance [30].

SSBs, especially those high in fructose, are known to induce glomerular hyperfiltration, which contributes significantly to a decline in kidney function [30]. Fructose intake has been shown to initiate inflammatory responses, induce oxidative stress, and alter the composition of gut microbiota [30]. Moreover, both sugar-sweetened and artificially sweetened beverages are rich in phosphorus and dietary acid, which are recognized as risk factors for kidney disease [30].

In this regard, abnormal metabolic status such as imbalance of glucose metabolism, acid-base metabolism, and more severe inflammatory status compared to the general population has been shown in CKD patients [32]. This issue makes it difficult to explain the clear effects of SSB consumption on physiological and pathophysiological processes, but it may be considered a factor for creating a vicious cycle and increasing mortality due to unbalanced metabolism [32]. In this regard, it has been shown that SSB consumption leads to visceral adiposity and low-grade inflammation due to its high sugar content and zero nutrients [33]. Therefore, high consumption of SSB plays an important role in adiposity, diabetes, and inflammation [33]. Visceral adipose tissue plays an important role in the production of adipokines as cytokines secreted from adipose tissue that are strongly related to the increase in the level of inflammatory biomarkers [33]. On the other hand, the accumulation of excess fat in the liver and adipose tissue following the consumption of excess sugar leads to the release of free fatty acids, which by inhibiting insulin-stimulated glucose metabolism leads to insulin resistance [33]. So, these mechanisms refer to kidney dysfunction and make it harder to control following the increase in SSB consumption [32].

According to recent findings, chronic consumption of sugary drinks has been linked to mitochondria changes of skeletal muscles that impair muscle strength [28]. Branganca et al.'s study also reported that daily consumption of SSBs leads to a decrease in muscle mass index [34]. Furthermore, Hao et al. reported that the consumption of SSBs decreases muscle mass [35]. On the other hand, the consumption of SSBs is associated with increased muscle fat, which stimulates muscle lipolysis and autophagy, and decreases myogenesis and muscle mass [36–39]. Finally, the consumption of SSBs leads to a loss of muscle mass and, thus, an increased risk of sarcopenia. This occurs through effects on glucose and lipid metabolism, reduced protein synthesis, and decreased efficiency of muscle contraction [36–39].

9. Ultra-processed foods (UPFs) and sarcopenia

In Iran, there is an increasing tendency to consume hydrogenated fats, animal fats, products containing sugar, packaged snacks, low-fiber foods, artificially sweetened beverages, and processed foods [40]. As a result, the concept of nutrition transition is becoming significantly more pronounced [40]. As a result, the modern dietary patterns have replaced those of the traditional diet [40].

UPFs are defined as ready-to-heat or ready-to-eat foods [40] that contain high levels of free sugars, saturated fats, salt, phosphorus, energy, and additives, and low levels of micronutrients, fiber content, and protein [40, 41]. The consumption of UPFs has significantly increased in previous years and has replaced the consumption of healthy foods, such as fruits, vegetables, legumes, and nuts [41]. According to epidemiological findings, UPFs are harmful to health [40] and they are associated with an increased risk of chronic disorders [42]. Therefore, dietary guidelines recommend eliminating the use of UPFs and reducing the consumption of processed foods [42]. Sarcopenic subjects have been reported to be more exposed to UPFs compared to non-sarcopenic subjects [43]. Sandoval-Insausti et al. have shown a strong relationship between UPF consumption and frailty risk in the elderly [44]. Zhang et al. also reported that UPFs intake in the elderly decreased muscle strength [45]. UPF intake is associated with poor diet quality, leading to reduced intake of fiber, fruits, vegetables, and protein and increased intake of energy-dense and nutritionally deficient foods [43]. This dietary pattern is related to the decrease in muscle mass in the elderly and the exacerbation of sarcopenia [43].

A positive association has been reported between UPF intake and the risk of CKD disease. Production of UPFs is associated with chemical reactions, the addition of various additives, and complex packaging [46]. These processes are known as factors related in the occurrence of CKD [46]. Glycosylation end products (AGEs) produced during food processing are important due to Millard reactions [46]. AGEs play a role in glomerulosclerosis, basement membrane thickening, and tubulointerstitial fibrosis, contributing in kidney damage [46]. Sodium benzoate (SB), potassium sorbate (PS), monosodium glutamate (MSG), and butylated hydroxytoluene are used as food preservatives in UPF. These preservatives increase the shelf life of food and prevent bacterial infections [46]. As shown in an animal study, exposure to SB and PS was associated with a significant increase in urea, creatinine, uric acid levels, and indicators of kidney damage [47].

Consuming UPFs is associated with the intake of high amounts of energy, saturated and trans fatty acids, sugar, and salt. Excessive consumption of energy and sugar is associated with obesity, which is recognized as a major contributor to the development of CKD [46]. Moreover, excessive consumption of fructose leads to damage in the glomerular interstitial and vascular arteriopathy. It also increases the level of uric acid, which acts as a pro-inflammatory and pro-oxidant factor for kidney tissue, causing damage to the kidney microvasculature and glomerulus [46]. On the other hand, UPFs are poor in protein, vitamins, minerals, and other phytochemicals, all of which are essential nutrients for muscle health [40].

In Shateri et al.'s study, the relationship between higher consumption of UPFs and sarcopenia in CKD patients was reported [40]. Several factors such as insulin resistance, acidosis, vitamin D deficiency, and hormonal disorders (e.g., testosterone, IGF-1, and growth hormone) are recognized as etiological factors contributing to the development of sarcopenia in CKD patients. These factors are exacerbated by the consumption of UPFs [40]. Exposure to phthalates as a result of food processing plastics or leakage in content with the material can alter the gut microbiome or disrupt gut barrier function, leading to inflammatory conditions [40]. These inflammatory conditions are known to be important factors in muscle wasting [40]. The findings also reported the relationship between exposure to phthalates and lower grip strength, a marker of muscle health and sarcopenia [40, 48]. Moreover, inadequate fiber intake causes the accumulation of protein fermentation metabolites, uremic toxicity, and, ultimately, uremic muscle wasting [40].

10. Conclusions

In summary, this research indicates that high consumption of SSBs and UPFs can significantly enhance the achievement of low muscle strength and increase the risk of sarcopenia. Also, this research contributes to the expanding body of literature that underscores the importance of dietary factors in muscle strength and sarcopenia. The intake of SSBs and UPFs, coupled with poor diet quality and inadequate nutrient-dense foods, may increase the risk or exacerbate sarcopenia in older adult CKD patients. As the population ages, preventing sarcopenia becomes vital for enhancing the quality of life for individuals as they spend more time in their senior years. Further research is needed to fully comprehend the mechanisms behind the observed associations and to clarify the role of diet in preventing sarcopenia.

Author details

Marzieh Mahmoodi[1,2], Fatemeh Mansouri[2], Maede Makhtoomi[1,3], Zainab Shateri[4] and Mehran Nouri[3,5*]

1 Student Research Committee, Shiraz University of Medical Sciences, Shiraz, Iran

2 Department of Clinical Nutrition, School of Nutrition and Food Sciences, Shiraz University of Medical Sciences, Shiraz, Iran

3 Health Policy Research Center, Institute of Health, Shiraz University of Medical Sciences, Shiraz, Iran

4 Department of Nutrition and Biochemistry, School of Medicine, Ilam University of Medical Sciences, Ilam, Iran

5 Mobility Impairment Research Center, Health Research Institute, Babol University of Medical Sciences, Babol, Iran

*Address all correspondence to: mehran_nouri71@yahoo.com

References

[1] Mallamaci F, Tripepi G. Risk factors of chronic kidney disease progression: Between old and new concepts. Journal of Clinical Medicine. 2024;**13**(3):678

[2] Kovesdy CP. Epidemiology of chronic kidney disease: An update 2022. Kidney International Supplements. 2022;**12**(1):7-11

[3] Mills KT et al. A systematic analysis of worldwide population-based data on the global burden of chronic kidney disease in 2010. Kidney International. 2015;**88**(5):950-957

[4] Hill NR et al. Global prevalence of chronic kidney disease–a systematic review and meta-analysis. PLoS One. 2016;**11**(7):e0158765

[5] Kazancioğlu R. Risk factors for chronic kidney disease: An update. Kidney International Supplements. 2013;**3**(4):368-371

[6] Chatzipetrou V et al. Sarcopenia in chronic kidney disease: A scoping review of prevalence, risk factors, association with outcomes, and treatment. Calcified Tissue International. 2022;**110**(1):1-31

[7] Damluji AA et al. Sarcopenia and cardiovascular diseases. Circulation. 2023;**147**(20):1534-1553

[8] Ramadas A et al. Diet quality and measures of sarcopenia in developing economies: A systematic review. Nutrients. 2022;**14**(4):868

[9] Mahmoodi M et al. The association between healthy beverage index and sarcopenia in Iranian older adults: A case-control study. BMC Geriatrics. 2024;**24**(1):244

[10] Mahmoodi M et al. Association between oxidative balance score and sarcopenia in older adults. Scientific Reports. 2024;**14**(1):5362

[11] Beaudart C et al. Sarcopenia and health-related quality of life: A systematic review and meta-analysis. Journal of Cachexia, Sarcopenia and Muscle. 2023;**14**(3):1228-1243

[12] Pascual-Fernández J et al. Sarcopenia: Molecular pathways and potential targets for intervention. International Journal of Molecular Sciences. 2020;**21**(22):8844

[13] Fielding RA et al. Sarcopenia: An undiagnosed condition in older adults. Current consensus definition: Prevalence, etiology, and consequences. International working group on sarcopenia. Journal of the American Medical Directors Association. 2011;**12**(4):249-256

[14] Sieber CC. Malnutrition and sarcopenia. Aging Clinical and Experimental Research. 2019;**31**(6):793-798

[15] Smith C et al. Sarcopenia definition: Does it really matter? Implications for resistance training. Ageing Research Reviews. 2022;**78**:101617

[16] Cruz-Jentoft AJ et al. Sarcopenia: Revised European consensus on definition and diagnosis. Age and Ageing. 2019;**48**(1):16-31

[17] Gungor O et al. Effects of hormonal changes on sarcopenia in chronic kidney disease: Where are we now and what can we do? Journal of Cachexia, Sarcopenia and Muscle. 2021;**12**(6):1380-1392

[18] Zupo R et al. Ultra-processed food consumption and nutritional

frailty in older age. Geroscience. 2023;**45**(4):2229-2243

[19] Robinson S, Cooper C, Aihie Sayer A. Nutrition and sarcopenia: A review of the evidence and implications for preventive strategies. Journal of Aging Research. 2012;**2012**:510801

[20] Papadopoulou SK et al. Mediterranean diet and sarcopenia features in apparently healthy adults over 65 years: A systematic review. Nutrients. 2023;**15**(5):1104

[21] Massini G et al. Nutritional strategies to prevent muscle loss and sarcopenia in chronic kidney disease: What do we currently know? Nutrients. 2023;**15**(14):3107

[22] Inoshita H et al. Cross-sectional study on the association between dietary patterns and sarcopenia in elderly patients with chronic kidney disease receiving conservative treatment. Nutrients. 2023;**15**(23):4994

[23] Masot O et al. Fluid intake recommendation considering the physiological adaptations of adults over 65 years: A critical review. Nutrients. 2020;**12**(11):3383

[24] Dominguez LJ et al. Adherence to a healthy beverage score is associated with lower frailty risk in older adults. Nutrients. 2022;**14**(18):3861

[25] Struijk EA et al. Sweetened beverages and risk of frailty among older women in the Nurses' health study: A cohort study. PLoS Medicine. 2020;**17**(12):e1003453

[26] Ejtahed HS et al. Sugar-sweetened beverage consumption is associated with metabolic syndrome in Iranian adults: Tehran lipid and glucose study. Endocrinology and Metabolism (Seoul). 2015;**30**(3):334-342

[27] Mansouri M et al. Sugar-sweetened beverages consumption in relation to hypertension among Iranian university students: The MEPHASOUS study. Eating and Weight Disorders. 2020;**25**(4):973-982

[28] Zhang Y et al. Association between sugar-sweetened beverage consumption frequency and muscle strength: Results from a sample of Chinese adolescents. BMC Public Health. 2023;**23**(1):1010

[29] Laclaustra M et al. Prospective association between added sugars and frailty in older adults. The American Journal of Clinical Nutrition. 2018;**107**(5):772-779

[30] Heo GY et al. Sweetened beverage intake and incident chronic kidney disease in the UK biobank study. JAMA Network Open. 2024;**7**(2):e2356885

[31] Yuzbashian E et al. Sugar-sweetened beverage consumption and risk of incident chronic kidney disease: Tehran lipid and glucose study. Nephrology (Carlton). 2016;**21**(7):608-616

[32] Cai XY et al. Sugar-sweetened beverage consumption and mortality of chronic kidney disease: Results from the US National Health and nutrition examination survey, 1999-2014. Clinical Kidney Journal. 2022;**15**(4):718-726

[33] Lin WT et al. Sugar-sweetened beverages intake, abdominal obesity, and inflammation among US adults without and with prediabetes-an NHANES study. International Journal of Environmental Research and Public Health. 2022;**20**(1):681

[34] Bragança M et al. The frequency of daily consumption of sugar-sweetened beverages is associated with reduced muscle mass index in adolescents. Nutrients. 2022;**14**(22):4917

[35] Hao G et al. Associations between muscle mass, physical activity and dietary behaviour in adolescents. Pediatric Obesity. 2019;**14**(3):e12471

[36] Barzilay JI et al. Insulin resistance and inflammation as precursors of frailty: The cardiovascular health study. Archives of Internal Medicine. 2007;**167**(7):635-641

[37] Cleasby ME, Jamieson PM, Atherton PJ. Insulin resistance and sarcopenia: Mechanistic links between common co-morbidities. The Journal of Endocrinology. 2016;**229**(2):R67-R81

[38] Aeberli I et al. Low to moderate sugar-sweetened beverage consumption impairs glucose and lipid metabolism and promotes inflammation in healthy young men: A randomized controlled trial. The American Journal of Clinical Nutrition. 2011;**94**(2):479-485

[39] Sørensen LB et al. Effect of sucrose on inflammatory markers in overweight humans. The American Journal of Clinical Nutrition. 2005;**82**(2):421-427

[40] Shateri Z et al. The role of ultra-processed food consumption in protein-energy wasting and sarcopenia development in patients with chronic kidney diseases. BMC Nephrology. 2024;**25**(1):4

[41] Mehrabani S et al. Consumption of ultra-processed foods could influence the metabolic syndrome odds: A cross-sectional study. Food Science & Nutrition. 2024;**12**(4):2567-2577

[42] Haghighatdoost F et al. Association between ultra-processed foods consumption and micronutrient intake and diet quality in Iranian adults: A multicentric study. Public Health Nutrition. 2022:1-9 [Preprint]

[43] Hao J, Zhou P, Qiu H. Association between ultra-processed food consumption and frailty in American elder people: Evidence from a cross-sectional study. The Journal of Nutrition, Health & Aging. 2022;**26**(7):688-697

[44] Sandoval-Insausti H et al. Ultra-processed food consumption and incident frailty: A prospective cohort study of older adults. The Journals of Gerontology. Series A, Biological Sciences and Medical Sciences. 2020;**75**(6):1126-1133

[45] Zhang S et al. Ultra-processed food intake is associated with grip strength decline in middle-aged and older adults: A prospective analysis of the TCLSIH study. European Journal of Nutrition. 2022;**61**(3):1331-1341

[46] Xiao B et al. Ultra-processed food consumption and the risk of incident chronic kidney disease: A systematic review and meta-analysis of cohort studies. Renal Failure. 2024;**46**(1):2306224

[47] Abd-Elhakim YM et al. Toll-like receptors and nuclear factor kappa B signaling pathway involvement in hepatorenal oxidative damage induced by some food preservatives in rats. Scientific Reports. 2023;**13**(1):5938

[48] Sun L et al. Exposure to phthalates is associated with grip strength in US adults. Ecotoxicology and Environmental Safety. 2021;**209**:111787

Section 2

Technologies and Methods for Neuromuscular Assessment

Chapter 6

Corticomuscular Coherence as Neurorehabilitation Assessment

Shun Sawai, Shoya Fujikawa, Ryosuke Yamamoto, Yusuke Shizuka, Naoki Shimizu, Kotaro Nakagawa and Hideki Nakano

Abstract

Corticomuscular coherence (CMC) is the correlation between electroencephalography (EEG), magnetoencephalography (MEG), and electromyography (EMG) and is a neurophysiological indicator that reflects functional connectivity between the brain and muscle. This indicator includes both descending (such as motor commands) and ascending (such as sensory inputs) information transmission. Therefore, the relationship between motor control and CMC and changes in CMC due to motor learning were examined. During neurorehabilitation, interventions often aim to promote motor learning and acquire motor control, making CMC a useful tool in neurorehabilitation. This review provides an overview of CMC based on basic and applied clinical research, facilitating its use as a neurophysiological assessment method for neurorehabilitation.

Keywords: corticomuscular coherence, motor control, motor learning, neurorehabilitation, physical therapy, assessment

1. Introduction

Coherence refers to the degree of consistency or relevance between different data elements or information in data analysis and processing, often used in optics and physics, indicating consistent wave properties or phases [1]. *In vivo* coherence is used in electroencephalography (EEG) [2] and electromyography (EMG) [3]. In EEG, coherence between two electrodes reflects the transfer of information in the brain [4]. In EMG, coherence between two electrodes within one muscle or between two muscles is used to quantify common oscillatory input to motor neurons within a frequency band [5], assessing whether the muscles work in concert. Therefore, coherence is used to analyze electrical signals *in vivo*.

Corticomuscular coherence (CMC) is the coherence between EMG and EEG, which is an evaluation index reflecting the functional connectivity between cortical activity and muscles (**Figure 1**) [6, 7]. This correlation evaluates both motor

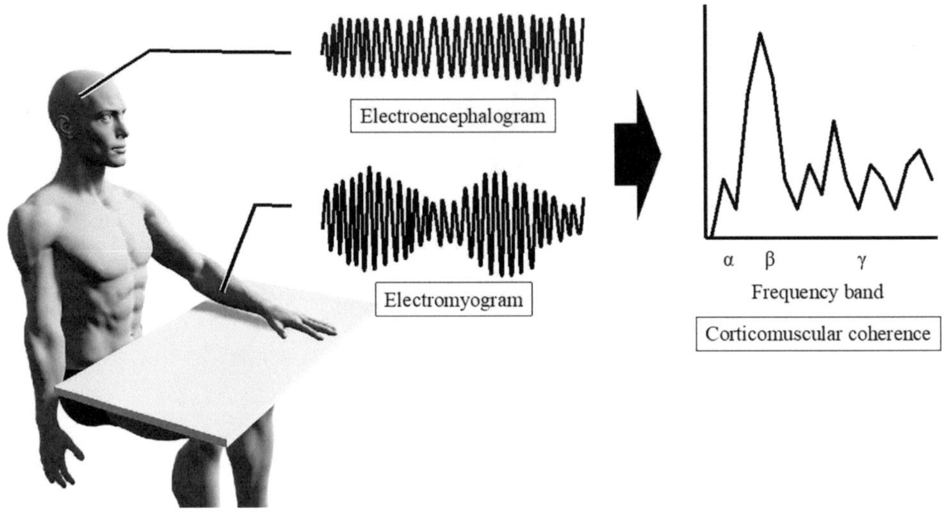

Figure 1.
Corticomuscular coherence. EEG and EMG are measured, and the value of CMC is calculated for each frequency band. The CMC in the β and γ frequency bands increases during exercise [6].

commands from the brain to muscles and sensory feedback from muscles to the brain [8]. Conventional brain and muscle functional assessments alone are limited to brain and muscle evaluations. In contrast, CMC is a comprehensive evaluation index that includes both brain and muscle elements from central to peripheral regions. Therefore, CMC can be used to elucidate motor control, motor learning mechanisms, and the pathophysiology of neurological diseases.

CMC is calculated using the following equation [7]:

$$CMC(f) = \frac{\left|PS_{S1,S2}(f)\right|^2}{\left|PS_{S1}(f)\right|\left|PS_{S2}(f)\right|} \quad (1)$$

Here, f refers to an arbitrary frequency band, and $PS_{S1}(f)$ and $PS_{S2}(f)$ are the spectral power values of the EMG and EEG or magnetoencephalography (MEG) data, respectively. $PS_{S1,S2}(f)$ represent the cross-spectrum values between the EMG and EEG or MEG data. The value of CMC ranges from 0 to 1, with 1 indicating an ideal correlation between the two signals and 0 indicating no association. Therefore, a high CMC indicates high functional connectivity between the brain and muscle and is a comprehensive neurophysiological evaluation index from the center to the periphery.

In this chapter, CMC, as an evaluation index in neurorehabilitation, is reviewed based on basic research on healthy participants and clinical studies on patients with neurological diseases and other disorders.

2. Basic research on CMC

CMC is a neurophysiological measure used for evaluating motor control and examining the effects of motor learning. This section describes CMC based on studies involving healthy participants.

2.1 CMC as an assessment measure for motor control

Improving motor control is the primary goal of rehabilitation, especially in neurological diseases such as stroke [9]. Motor control is evaluated using kinematic parameters (velocity and acceleration of movement), kinetic parameters (force and torque), and physiological parameters (such as EMG) [10]. Additionally, many neural mechanisms related to motor control have been verified, and the primary motor cortex, other motor-related areas [11], and the basal ganglia [12] and cerebellum [13] are involved in motor control. Furthermore, both the brain and spinal cord are significantly involved in motor control [14]. These neural mechanisms have been elucidated by measuring the neural activity during motor control using EEG, functional near-infrared spectroscopy, and functional magnetic resonance imaging. However, most conventional evaluation methods target only the brain. A method for evaluating the excitability of the corticospinal tract involves using transcranial magnetic stimulation (TMS) as a comprehensive index from the brain to the periphery [15]. In addition to TMS, CMC is used as a comprehensive neurological evaluation index for motor control from the brain to the periphery.

Many studies have shown the effectiveness of CMC in motor control tasks requiring steady motor output [16]. These tasks involve maintaining a constant force, such as holding the fingers at 10 or 30% of the maximum force or gripping and holding the fingers in a fixed position against external forces [17–19]. Kristeva et al. [17] examined CMC in the sensorimotor region and beta frequency band (15–30 Hz), while participants held their fingers in a fixed position against an external force of 4% maximal contraction on the right index finger flexor muscle. The results showed that the CMC in the beta frequency band was significantly higher in participants who could maintain a constant position against an external force than in those who could not. This frequency band has been linked to attention [20], suggesting that more focused participants performed better on this task, which may have affected their CMC. CMC involves sensorimotor integration, encompassing both descending motor and ascending sensory information, indicating its potential role in motor control performance, which relies on motor-sensory regulation in the cerebral cortex and cerebellum [21].

Furthermore, the relationship between motor control and CMC is becoming clearer not only for simple hand tasks but also for whole-body movements. Kenville et al. [22] measured EEG and EMG during a bipedal squat movement and examined CMC during each phase of the movement (**Figure 2**). The squat phase consisted of an eccentric phase in which the center of gravity was lowered from the standing position, an isometric phase in which the center of gravity was held low, and a concentric phase in which the center of gravity was raised to the standing position. In this study, the EMG was derived from the vastus lateralis, vastus medialis, tibialis anterior, and erector spinae muscles. EEG was derived from 32 electrodes that were set up to cover the bilateral primary motor cortices. The results showed that CMCs in the β (13–30 Hz) and γ (30–44 Hz) frequency bands were significantly higher in the eccentric and concentric phases than in the isometric phase. This suggests that CMCs in the β and γ frequency bands may be involved in movement control. Thus, CMCs were observed in isometric and isotonic movements, possibly clarifying how the brain and muscles are functionally and differentially connected to control movements depending on the movement style. In this study, partially directed coherence analysis was used to verify directional CMC, which included both ascending and descending signals. The results showed that the EMG-to-EEG connectivity was higher in

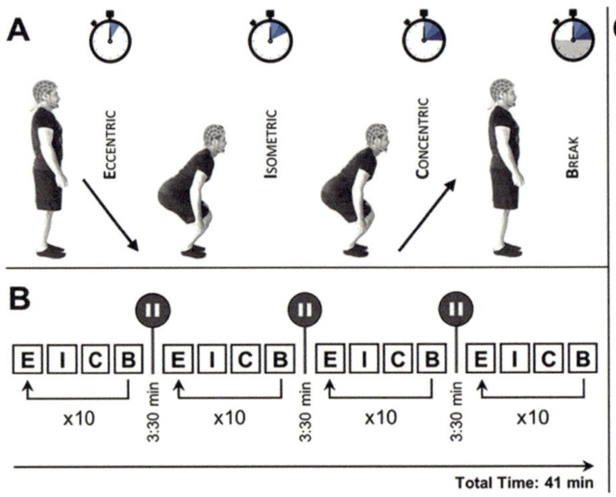

Figure 2.
CMC during the bipedal squat [22]. (A, B) The bipedal squat was divided into four periods, and CMC was calculated at each period. (C) The EEG was derived from 32 electrodes around the bilateral primary motor cortex.

the eccentric phase, and the EEG-to-EMG connectivity was higher in the concentric phase. This can be explained by the fact that centrifugal contraction depends on afferent information *via* the muscle spindles [23].

Thus, CMC is related to motor control performance and can evaluate the state of brain-muscle communication using motor control. Therefore, CMC may be used as a detailed evaluation index for motor control during neurorehabilitation.

2.2 CMC as an assessment measure for motor learning

Motor learning is a process related to practice and experience, which leads to permanent changes in the ability to perform proficiently [24]. Motor learning has been proposed as a background mechanism for functional improvement in neurorehabilitation [25, 26], and new neurorehabilitation techniques, such as robotic rehabilitation, have been developed based on the motor learning theory [27]. Motor learning produces changes at the behavioral and neurological levels, and its effects and mechanisms have been examined using behavioral indices, muscle activity evaluation, and neural activity evaluation [28]. However, these evaluation indices evaluate the muscles or brain alone, and evaluating the entire body as a neural system from the brain to the muscles is impossible.

CMC has been used to assess the effects of motor learning. Several studies have shown that motor learning increases CMC; however, some studies report varying changes among individuals [29, 30]. Perez et al. [29] performed a visuomotor task using foot movements and compared CMC with the activity of the primary motor cortex involved in foot movements and the tibialis anterior muscle before and after the task. The task required participants to move their ankle joints to a specified angle according to a diagram projected on a computer monitor. The participants were divided into two groups: one with visual feedback on their ankle joint angles and the other without visual feedback. The results showed that motor learning was more effective in the group with visual feedback than in the group without visual feedback, and CMC in the beta frequency band (15–35 Hz) in the group with visual feedback increased significantly after motor learning. CMC is mediated by fast corticospinal axons and monosynaptic connections to spinal motor neurons [5]. Motor learning tasks cause increased cortical excitability in the primary motor cortex [30], indicating that increased excitability in the corticospinal tract may result in a higher CMC. Thus, motor learning increases CMC. However, some reports indicate individual differences in CMC changes owing to motor learning [31]. Mendez-Balbuena et al. [31] performed a visuomotor learning task requiring constant index finger force control and compared the CMC before and after motor learning. The results showed that CMC in the beta (15–31 Hz) and gamma (31–45 Hz) frequency bands significantly increased before and after the visuomotor learning task. However, an additional analysis divided the participants into two groups: one where significant CMCs were generated during the baseline task before learning and the other in which no significant CMCs were generated during the task before learning. Furthermore, the group where significant CMCs were generated before learning exhibited greater motor learning effects. CMCs, mainly in the γ frequency band, are involved in centrifugal neurotransmission, afferent sensory information transmission, and sensory integration [32]. Therefore, participants who had significant CMC before learning experienced sensory integration during exercise, and motor learning may have further promoted sensory integration and enhanced the learning effect. Although CMC increases with motor learning, individual differences exist in the values and amounts of change.

Consequently, motor learning increases CMC, which forms the scientific basis for neurorehabilitation. In particular, because CMC is an index that includes centrifugal neurotransmission and integrates afferent sensory information, it encompasses the entire mechanism of motor learning theory and may be widely used in the future as a neurological index that reflects the effects of motor learning.

2.3 Summary

This section reviews basic research on CMC and its use as an assessment index for motor control and learning. Research on healthy participants shows that high motor control performance is associated with high CMC values. CMC also increases as motor learning progresses. Since motor control and learning involve both centrifugal motor commands and afferent sensory information integration, CMC likely reflects the communication between the brain and muscles. These processes are crucial for both neurorehabilitation and general rehabilitation. Therefore, CMC has potential as a future evaluation index for neurorehabilitation.

3. Applied research on CMC

CMC has been validated for motor control and learning in healthy participants, older adults, and patients with neurological diseases, making it a potential evaluation index for neurorehabilitation. This section describes CMC based on clinical research in older adults and patients with neurological diseases, offering insights into its application for neurorehabilitation.

3.1 CMC as a functional assessment of aging

Physical [33] and cognitive [34] functions decline with aging, and an accurate understanding of functional decline and effective interventions against it have been studied from various aspects [35, 36]. In addition, a decline in physical function involves both muscle and brain function [37, 38]. Therefore, EEG and noninvasive brain stimulation methods have been used to evaluate brain function in older adults compared to younger adults and to verify changes in brain function with aging [39]. In this context, the resting EEG [40], resting brain connectivity [41, 42], and EEG signals during mental activity [43] change with age. Furthermore, EEG stability and functional connectivity decrease, whereas activity increases in some brain regions. In addition to evaluating the brain alone, CMC has shown potential for use as a comprehensive evaluation index for muscles in older adults.

Several studies have reported that CMC increases with age [44, 45]. Kemp et al. [44] performed a task to maintain muscle output at 20% of the maximal contraction during isometric contraction of the right forearm and compared the CMC of the extensor digitorum muscle and primary motor cortex in young and older adults during this task. In this study, we used MEG to measure brain function. The results showed that the CMC amplitude in the beta frequency band (13–30 Hz) was significantly higher in older adults than in younger adults. In addition, the power of the primary motor cortex decreased, whereas that of the extensor digitorum muscle and CMC increased in older adults. This increase in CMC may represent a compensatory mechanism and prevent the decline in function by increasing neural resources and enhancing cortical-muscle connectivity. This result is consistent with brain overactivity in older adults, as shown in fMRI studies [46], indicating that more neural resources are expended to control movement.

In contrast, CMC is lower in older adults than in younger adults [47–49]. Yoshida et al. [47] examined the changes in CMC between the tibialis anterior and medial gastrocnemius muscles and the primary motor cortex of the foot region during externally paced, periodic, and counter-phase plantar dorsiflexion exercises in the sitting position in young and older adults. In other words, this task implies movement such that the right foot dorsiflexes and the left foot plantarflexes. The results showed significant CMCs in the tibialis anterior muscle and primary motor cortex in both young and older adults. However, a significant CMC of the medial gastrocnemius muscle was more prevalent in younger adults than in older adults (**Figure 3**). The CMC of older adults was significantly lower than that of younger adults. Furthermore, a lower CMC in the elderly was unrelated to their performance in plantar dorsiflexion exercises. This indicates that CMC declines prior to the level at which motor performance declines, suggesting that CMC may be used as a predictor of age-related decline in physical function. This study indicates that increased activity in the spinal cord and other areas outside the cortex owing to periodic exercise may cause low CMC in older adults; however, further research is needed to identify the cause based on neuroscientific findings.

Thus, changes in CMC with age did not yield consistent results. Other neurological studies support the hypothesis that CMC increases with age as older adults maintain compensatory performance by expending more neural resources. However, because coherence in the brain declines with age [41, 42], we cannot rule out the possibility that functional connectivity is impaired with age, not only within the brain but also between the brain and muscle. Future studies should examine these mechanisms in more detail to clarify how CMCs change with aging and how they can be used as indicators to assess aging.

3.2 CMC as a functional assessment for patients with stroke

Stroke is a neurological disease that causes motor paralysis, sensory impairment, and higher brain dysfunction, depending on the site of onset [50, 51]. Stroke causes significant loss of motor control, and neurorehabilitation is used to reacquire

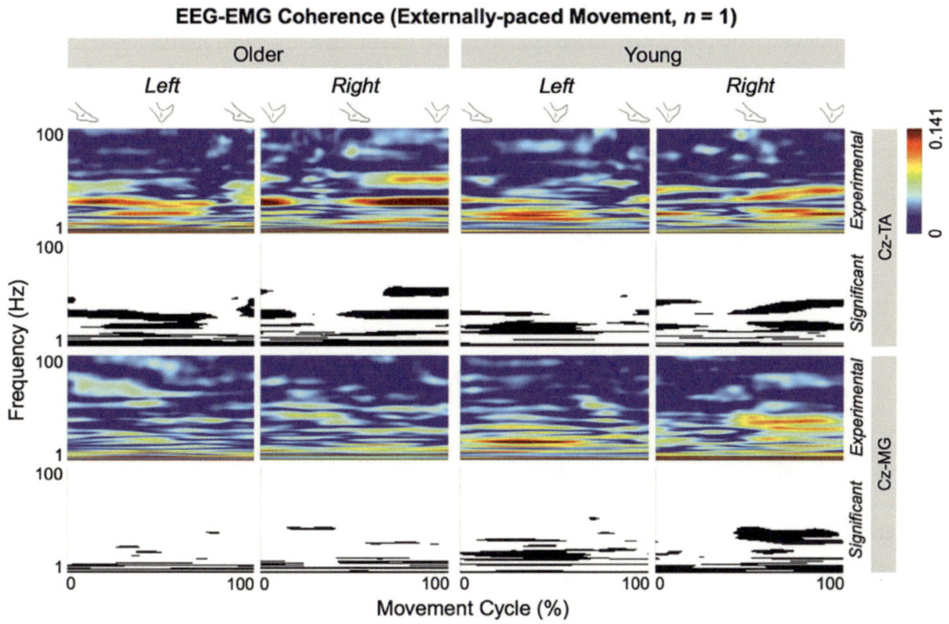

Figure 3.
CMC during plantar dorsiflexion exercise in young and older adults [47]. Significant CMC of the tibialis anterior muscle and primary motor cortex were identified during all periods of plantar dorsiflexion exercise in both young and older adults. In contrast, significant CMC of the medial gastrocnemius and primary motor cortex was found only in younger adults.

function [52]. Behavioral [53, 54] and neurological indices have been used to evaluate the severity of functional impairment due to stroke and the degree of recovery by rehabilitation [55]. In particular, EEG [56] and TMS [57] have been used as neurological measures, and evaluations have been conducted in the brain and throughout the corticospinal tract. CMC, like TMS, can evaluate brain and muscle functions and may be used to evaluate stroke severity and the recovery process.

CMC has been consistently shown to decrease during the acute phase of stroke [58–60]. Furthermore, CMC increases with recovery and approaches normal state [61, 62]. Krauth et al. [61] continuously measured CMC in the beta frequency band (12–30 Hz) during simultaneous bilateral wrist dorsiflexion movements in patients with left-sided stroke at three-time points to examine the changes in CMC from stroke onset to recovery. In this study, the EMG was derived from the right wrist extensor, and the EEG was derived from all brain regions at 60 ch according to the international 10-10 method. Fugl-Meyer assessment for behavioral data and EEG and EMG for neurophysiological data were performed at approximately 1–2 weeks, 7 weeks, and 6.5–15 months after onset. The results showed that healthy young adults had a CMC in the left primary motor cortex corresponding to right-hand movements (**Figure 4**), whereas patients with stroke had lower CMC in the left primary motor cortex than healthy young adults (**Figure 5**). Furthermore, after the onset of stroke, the area in which significant CMC was observed expanded, and the CMC value increased. In particular, the expansion of CMC during recovery is bilateral, aligning with neuroscientific evidence that surrounding areas mobilize after stroke [63], and it is highly likely that CMC reflects the neurological recovery process after stroke. Moreover, a significant positive correlation between the Fugl-Meyer assessment of

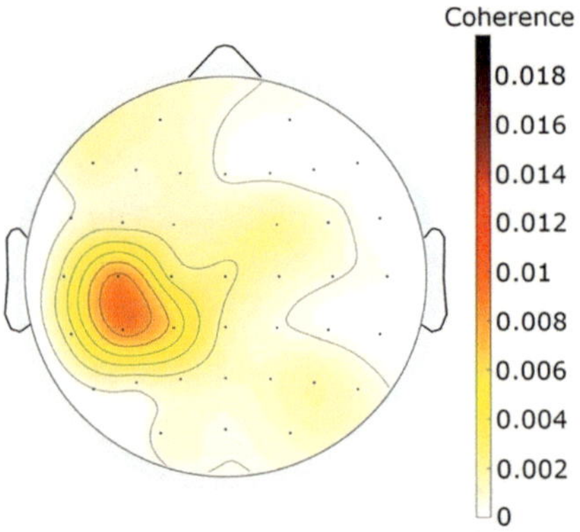

Figure 4.
CMC with the right wrist extensor during bilateral simultaneous wrist dorsiflexion movements in healthy young subjects [61]. The CMC is higher in the left primary motor cortex, corresponding to right-hand movements.

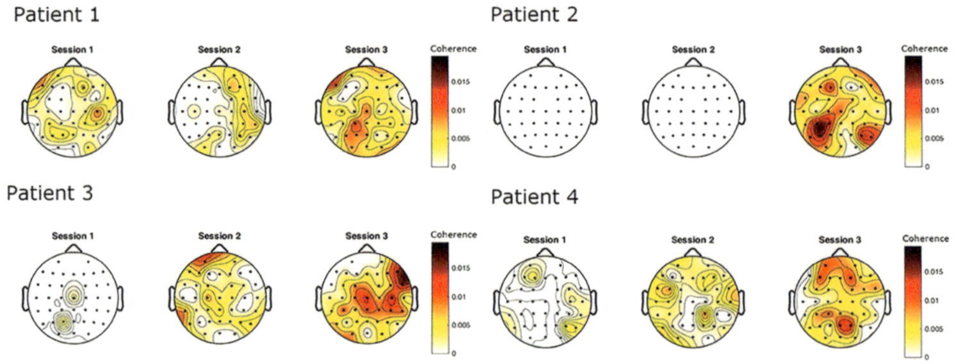

Figure 5.
Changes in CMC from onset to recovery in patients with stroke [61]. From the acute phase (session 1) to the chronic phase (session 3), the CMC increased in all four patients, and its observed range expanded. In addition, the CMC in the left primary motor cortex, which corresponds to right-hand movements, is lower than that in healthy young adults.

upper limb function and peak CMC (**Figure 6**) indicates that higher upper limb function corresponds to higher CMC, reflecting the disease status and recovery process of patients with upper limb dysfunction after stroke.

In addition to simple CMC, the neural mechanisms of motor control in patients with chronic stroke have been examined using temporal dynamic analysis of changes in CMC during isotonic movements [64]. Temporal changes in CMC during elbow extension movements were compared between healthy participants and patients with stroke. In this study, the EMG was derived from the biceps brachii, triceps brachii, brachioradialis, and brachioradialis muscles. EEG signals were derived from C3 and C4, which correspond to the primary motor cortex. The results showed that the CMC between the triceps brachii, primary action muscle, and primary motor cortex was not significantly different between healthy participants and patients with stroke. However, the CMC in the beta frequency band (13–30 Hz) between the brachialis muscle, antagonist muscle, and primary motor cortex was significantly higher in patients with stroke than in healthy participants during the early phase of elbow extension (**Figure** 7). This high CMC in the beta frequency band (13–30 Hz)

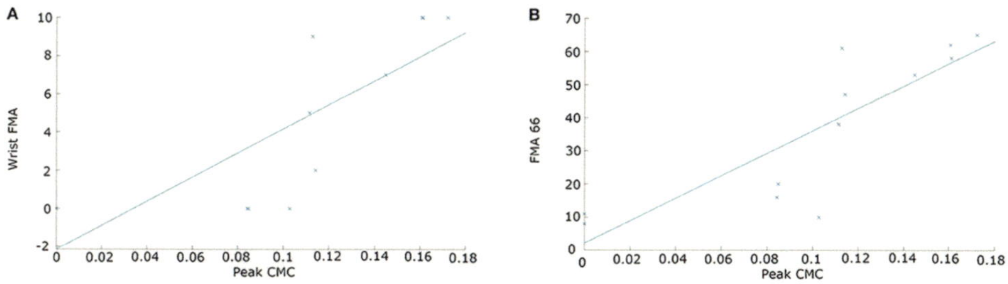

Figure 6.
Relationship between CMC and upper limb function [61]. A significant positive correlation between the Fugl-Meyer assessment of upper limb function and CMC has been reported, indicating that higher upper limb function corresponds with higher CMC.

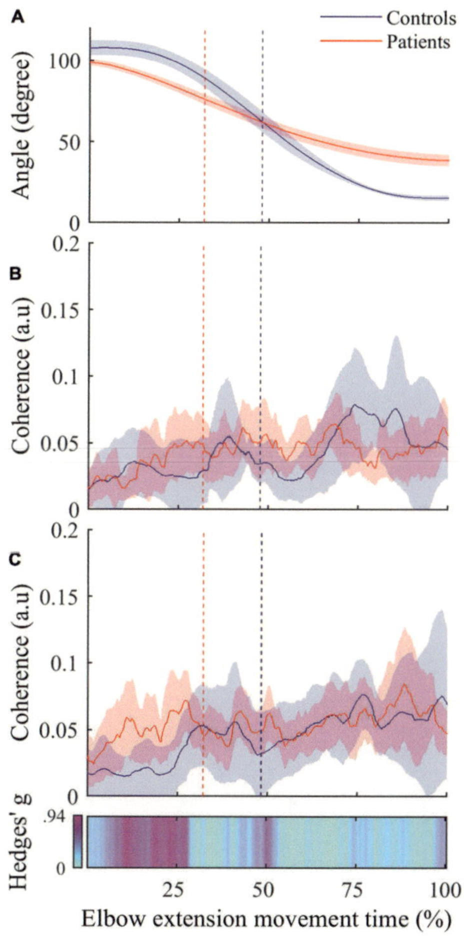

Figure 7.
Temporal changes in CMC during elbow extension exercise [64]. (A) Kinematic data of elbow extension in healthy participants and patients with stroke. The peak of acceleration is earlier in patients with stroke. (B) Temporal changes in the CMC of the triceps muscle and primary motor cortex. There was no significant difference in the CMC of the primary motor cortex between healthy participants and patients with stroke. (C) Temporal changes in the CMC of the antagonist brachialis muscle and primary motor cortex. "Hedges' g" indicates the effect size of the difference in CMC, 0 for cyan, and 0.94 for magenta. The CMC of the antagonist muscle in patients with stroke is higher than that of healthy participants in the early stage of elbow extension.

in the early motor phase in patients with stroke may be due to the increased afferent sensory input associated with movement and cooperative contraction of the primary and antagonist muscles owing to compensatory movements that differ from those of healthy participants. Motor commands are not transmitted to a single muscle but to other muscles during stroke [65], which may indicate a neurophysiological mechanism for this event. Thus, it is clear that CMC also differs in its changes and timing between patients with stroke and healthy participants, which could be used to understand motor control and its strategies in patients with stroke.

Furthermore, studies on patients with stroke show that CMC is influenced by pathological status, changes in physical function due to rehabilitation, and the actual study design (**Figure 8**) [66]. The brain region where CMC appears depends on the region where the stroke occurred [67], with some patients having a high CMC on the disabled side and others having a high CMC on the uninjured side. In addition, as mentioned above, CMC increases with recovery, which is another major factor affecting CMC. Moreover, repetitive functional training in rehabilitation causes cortical reorganization, which also affects CMC. Electrical stimulation used in rehabilitation has been shown to increase only the ascending CMC with weak stimulation, whereas strong stimulation increases both the ascending and descending CMCs [68]. Thus, CMC is altered by rehabilitation, which promotes cortical reorganization.

Thus, CMC in patients with stroke consistently decreases during the acute phase and increases with recovery. Rehabilitation-induced cortical reorganization may be involved in this trend, and CMC can be used to verify the effectiveness of neurorehabilitation. In addition, since spatial and temporal changes in CMC have been reported, CMC may be used to provide detailed neurophysiological outcomes of strokes.

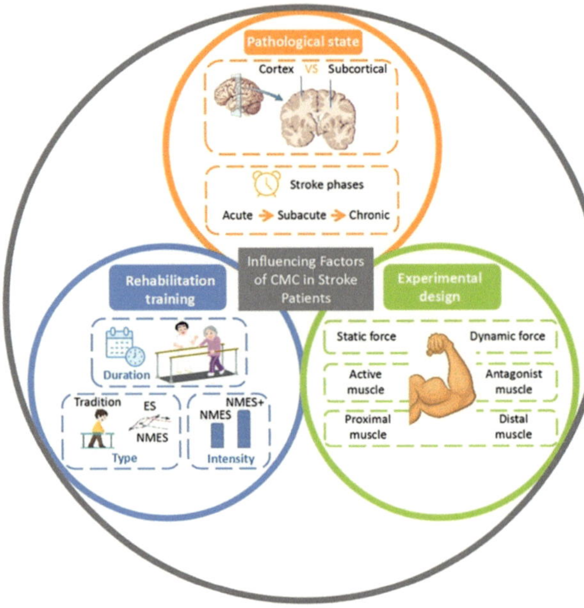

Figure 8.
Factors influencing CMC in patients with stroke [66]. In addition to pathological status, changes in physical function due to rehabilitation and the actual study design are factors influencing CMC in patients with stroke.

3.3 CMC as a functional assessment for patients with Parkinson's disease

Parkinson disease (PD) is a progressive neurodegenerative disease resulting from the pathophysiological loss or degeneration of dopaminergic neurons in the substantia nigra of the midbrain and the formation of Lewy bodies in neurons. PD is mainly characterized by stiffness, slow movement, and tremor [69, 70]. PD is known to cause difficulties in motor control owing to these symptoms [71], and neurorehabilitation is used to improve motor function. TMS [72] and EEG combined with TMS [73] have been used as neurophysiological evaluation indices for PD, and a comprehensive evaluation from brain to muscle has been developed. CMC, like TMS, is a comprehensive brain-to-muscle evaluation index that can be used to assess physical function, specific symptoms, and degree of disease progression in PD.

CMC is low in patients with PD during motor control, such as controlling the force exerted. Zokaei et al. [74] performed the task of gripping a device according to a specified force on healthy participants and patients with PD and examined the differences in CMC during the task (**Figure 9**). In this study, the EMG was derived from

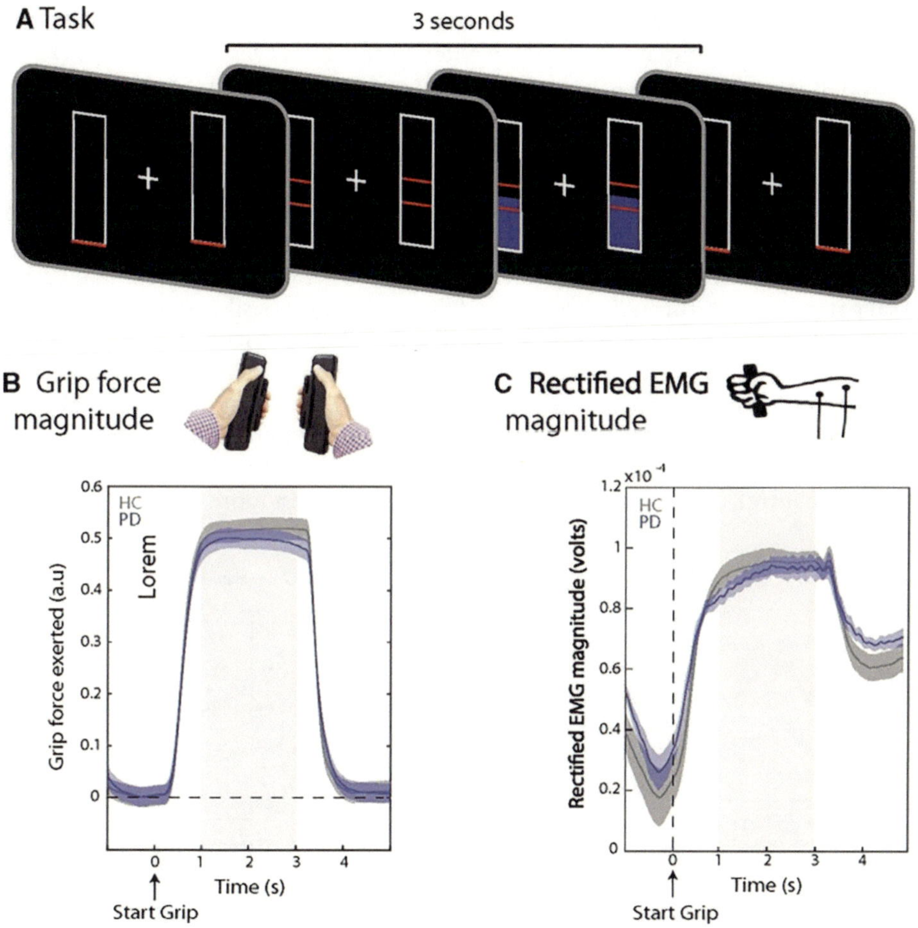

Figure 9.
Grip strength control task for patients with PD and healthy participants [74]. Participants performed the task of gripping the device with the indicated force based on visual feedback on the screen.

the bilateral flexor digitorum superficialis, and the MEG was derived from 306 ch in all brain regions. The results showed that CMCs were identified between the contralateral primary motor cortex and the flexor digitorum superficialis in both healthy participants and patients with PD. The CMC in the beta frequency band (11–25 Hz) was significantly higher in patients with PD than in healthy participants. Furthermore, a significant negative correlation was observed between motor item scores on the Unified Parkinson's Disease Rating Scale, a standard motor function measure in PD, and CMC in the beta frequency band (11–25 Hz) (**Figure 10**). These results indicate that CMC is reduced in patients with PD compared to healthy participants, suggesting that the more advanced the symptoms, the more pronounced the reduction in CMC. Deep brain stimulation has also been shown to reduce tremors and increase CMC in the active muscle and contralateral primary motor cortex [75]. In conclusion, there is a clear relationship between the CMC of patients with PD and their motor function, from both the perspective of brain function assessment and their response to brain stimulation.

In addition, patients with PD often experience gait disturbances owing to postural reflex impairment, and CMC has been used to examine the neural mechanisms of gait [76, 77]. However, the results are inconsistent. Yokoyama et al. [76] showed that the CMC in the beta frequency band (16–32 Hz) between the sensory-motor cortex and the tibialis anterior and medial gastrocnemius muscles was reduced during gait in patients with PD compared to healthy older adults. However, Roeder et al. [77] showed that the CMC in the lower beta frequency band (13–21 Hz) between the primary motor cortex and the tibialis anterior muscle was lower in healthy older adults and patients with PD than in healthy younger adults. However, there were no significant differences between healthy older adults and patients with PD. Unlike hand tasks, walking is a whole-body exercise in which several muscles and joints move cooperatively. Therefore, a CMC with a small number of muscles may not capture its characteristics. In addition, the walking rhythm is generated and regulated by the central pattern generator in the spinal cord [78], and it is possible that the CMC was not altered by processing in neural circuits distal to the cerebrum.

As described above, CMC may reflect the performance of motor control and severity of motor function in patients with PD, although, unlike stroke, the corticospinal tracts are not directly affected. CMC could be used as a new neurophysiological index for the neurorehabilitation of patients with PD. However, consistent results are limited to upper limb motor control, and further studies are required to assess more dynamic movements.

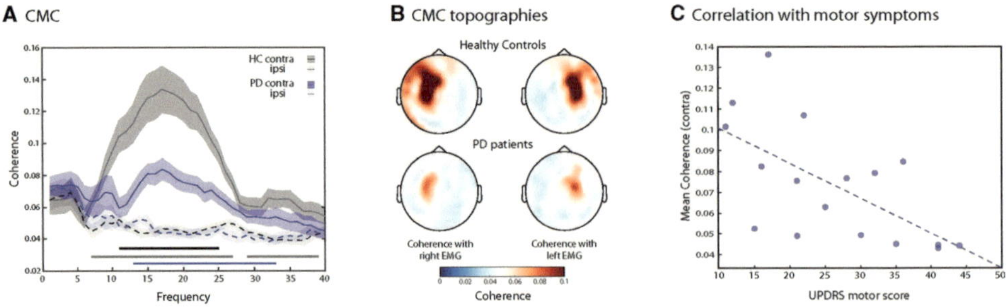

Figure 10.
CMC of healthy participants and patients with PD during a grip strength control task [74]. (A, B) Significantly lower CMC was found in patients with PD compared to healthy participants in the beta frequency band. (C) A significant negative correlation was observed between CMC and motor score on the Unified Parkinson's Disease Rating Scale, which indicates PD severity. This indicates that the lower the motor function, the lower the CMC in the beta frequency band.

3.4 CMC as a functional assessment for patients with development coordination disorder

Developmental coordination disorder (DCD) is a neurodevelopmental disorder affecting children's ability to perform coordinated motor actions, causing slow motor development, clumsiness, imprecision, and motor learning disabilities [79]. Therefore, neurorehabilitation should be performed in patients with DCD [80]. TMS has been widely used for neurophysiological assessment of motor function in patients with DCD [81]. Currently, patients with DCD have lower corticospinal tract excitability during motor imagery [82] and reduced online control of movement and inhibitory systems compared to healthy participants [83]. However, few studies have validated the use of CMC for motor control in patients with DCD, with only one case study conducted by Parr et al. [84]. They measured the CMC in the beta frequency band (15–35 Hz) between the shallow finger flexors and primary motor cortex during a force control task of wrist flexion in patients with DCD and healthy participants aged 34 and 29 years, respectively. The results showed that CMC was lower in patients with DCD than in healthy participants. This suggests that CMC can be used as a neurophysiological measure of motor control in patients with DCD. However, there are still many unknown factors owing to a lack of studies on patients with DCD. Therefore, further studies are needed to confirm this hypothesis. Further validation of neurorehabilitation in children with DCD will enable early and accurate evaluation of neurorehabilitation in children with DCD.

3.5 Summary

This section reviewed the application of CMC in neurorehabilitation based on clinical studies in older adults, patients with stroke, patients with PD, and patients with DCD. Older adults have a higher CMC during motor control than younger adults, suggesting that they may maintain their performance by compensatory overmobilization of the cortex. However, CMC is decreased in neurological diseases, such as stroke, PD, and DCD. Since CMC is related to the severity of the disease and the recovery process, it may be used as an evaluation index for the neurorehabilitation of neurological diseases. However, further research is needed to resolve the problems of inconsistent results and the small number of studies. With further research, CMC may become a standard neurophysiological assessment method for neurorehabilitation.

4. Conclusion

In this study, we reviewed CMC as a neurological evaluation index in neurorehabilitation based on studies involving both healthy participants and patients. Basic research has revealed that CMC is related to fundamental rehabilitation events, such as motor control and learning, and these findings have recently been applied to older adults and patients with neurological diseases. CMC is one of the few indices that encompasses the brain to the muscle and is useful because it includes descending information transmission, such as motor commands, and ascending information transmission, such as sensory input. Although CMC is still rarely used in actual rehabilitation practice, it may be used as an important neurophysiological index for understanding patient pathophysiology and verifying the effectiveness of rehabilitation as basic and clinical research continues to advance.

Acknowledgements

We would like to thank Editage (www.editage.com) for English language editing. This work was supported by JSPS KAKENHI (Grant Number JP23K10417) for HN and JSPS KAKENHI (Grant Number JP23K19907) for KN.

Conflict of interest

The authors declare no conflict of interest.

Appendices and nomenclature

EEG	electroencephalography
EMG	electromyography
CMC	corticomuscular coherence
MEG	magnetoencephalogram
PD	Parkinson's disease
DCD	developmental coordination disorder

Author details

Shun Sawai[1,2], Shoya Fujikawa[1,2], Ryosuke Yamamoto[1,3], Yusuke Shizuka[1,2], Naoki Shimizu[4], Kotaro Nakagawa[4,5] and Hideki Nakano[1,4*]

1 Neurorehabilitation Laboratory, Graduate School of Health Sciences, Kyoto Tachibana University, Kyoto, Japan

2 Department of Rehabilitation, Kyoto Kuno Hospital, Kyoto, Japan

3 Department of Rehabilitation, Tesseikai Neurosurgical Hospital, Osaka, Japan

4 Neurorehabilitation Laboratory, Department of Physical Therapy, Faculty of Health Sciences, Kyoto Tachibana University, Kyoto, Japan

5 Department of Rehabilitation, Nagashima Neurosurgery Rehabilitation Clinic, Osaka, Japan

*Address all correspondence to: nakano-h@tachibana-u.ac.jp

References

[1] Strömberg G. Coherence in the physical world. Philosophy of Science. 1942;**9**:323-334. DOI: 10.1086/286779

[2] Ruchkin D. EEG coherence. International Journal of Psychophysiology. 2005;**57**:83-85. DOI: 10.1016/j.ijpsycho.2005.04.001

[3] Dideriksen JL, Negro F, Falla D, Kristensen SR, Mrachacz-Kersting N, Farina D. Coherence of the surface EMG and common synaptic input to motor neurons. Frontiers in Human Neuroscience. 2018;**12**:207. DOI: 10.3389/fnhum.2018.00207

[4] Hallett M. EEG coherence: An introduction. Journal of Clinical Neurophysiology. 1999;**16**:499-500. DOI: 10.1097/00004691-199911000-00001

[5] Farmer SF, Bremner FD, Halliday DM, Rosenberg JR, Stephens JA. The frequency content of common synaptic inputs to motoneurones studied during voluntary isometric contraction in man. The Journal of Physiology. 1993;**470**:127-155. DOI: 10.1113/jphysiol.1993.sp019851

[6] Liu J, Sheng Y, Liu H. Corticomuscular coherence and its applications: A review. Frontiers in Human Neuroscience. 2019;**13**:100. DOI: 10.3389/fnhum.2019.00100

[7] Mima T, Hallett M. Corticomuscular coherence: A review. Journal of Clinical Neurophysiology. 1999;**16**:501-511. DOI: 10.1097/00004691-199911000-00002

[8] Yang Y, Dewald JPA, van der Helm FCT, Schouten AC. Unveiling neural coupling within the sensorimotor system: Directionality and nonlinearity. European Journal of Neuroscience. 2018;**48**:2407-2415. DOI: 10.1111/ejn.13692

[9] Dobkin BH. Strategies for stroke rehabilitation. The Lancet Neurology. 2004;**3**:528-536. DOI: 10.1016/S1474-4422(04)00851-8

[10] Hirschfeld H. Motor control of every day motor tasks: Guidance for neurological rehabilitation. Physiology & Behavior. 2007;**92**:161-166. DOI: 10.1016/j.physbeh.2007.05.018

[11] Bhattacharjee S, Kashyap R, Abualait T, Annabel Chen SH, Yoo WK, Bashir S. The role of primary motor cortex: More than movement execution. Journal of Motor Behavior. 2021;**53**:258-274. DOI: 10.1080/00222895.2020.1738992

[12] Groenewegen HJ. The basal ganglia and motor control. Neural Plasticity. 2003;**10**:107-120. DOI: 10.1155/NP.2003.107

[13] D'Angelo E. Physiology of the cerebellum. Handbook of Clinical Neurology. 2018;**154**:85-108. DOI: 10.1016/B978-0-444-63956-1.00006-0

[14] Poppele R, Bosco G. Sophisticated spinal contributions to motor control. Trends in Neuroscience. 2003;**26**:269-276. DOI: 10.1016/S0166-2236(03)00073-0

[15] Petersen NT, Pyndt HS, Nielsen JB. Investigating human motor control by transcranial magnetic stimulation. Experimental Brain Research. 2003;**152**:1-16. DOI: 10.1007/s00221-003-1537-y

[16] Boonstra TW. The potential of corticomuscular and intermuscular coherence for research on human motor control. Frontiers in Human Neuroscience. 2013;**7**:855. DOI: 10.3389/fnhum.2013.00855

[17] Kristeva R, Patino L, Omlor W. Beta-range cortical motor spectral power and corticomuscular coherence as a mechanism for effective corticospinal interaction during steady-state motor output. NeuroImage. 2007;**36**:785-792. DOI: 10.1016/j.neuroimage.2007.03.025

[18] Chakarov V, Naranjo JR, Schulte-Mönting J, Omlor W, Huethe F, Kristeva R. Beta-range EEG-EMG coherence with isometric compensation for increasing modulated low-level forces. Journal of Neurophysiology. 2009;**102**:1115-1120. DOI: 10.1152/jn.91095.2008

[19] Chen S, Entakli J, Bonnard M, Berton E, De Graaf JB. Functional corticospinal projections from human supplementary motor area revealed by corticomuscular coherence during precise grip force control. PLoS One. 2013;**8**:e60291. DOI: 10.1371/journal.pone.0060291

[20] Kristeva-Feige R, Fritsch C, Timmer J, Lücking CH. Effects of attention and precision of exerted force on beta range EEG-EMG synchronization during a maintained motor contraction task. Clinical Neurophysiology. 2002;**113**:124-131. DOI: 10.1016/s1388-2457(01)00722-2

[21] Kawato M, Furukawa K, Suzuki R. A hierarchical neural-network model for control and learning of voluntary movement. Biological Cybernetics. 1987;**57**:169-185. DOI: 10.1007/BF00364149

[22] Kenville R, Maudrich T, Vidaurre C, Maudrich D, Villringer A, Nikulin VV, et al. Corticomuscular interactions during different movement periods in a multi-joint compound movement. Scientific Reports. 2020;**10**:5021. DOI: 10.1038/s41598-020-61909-z

[23] Nagamori A, Valero-Cuevas FJ, Finley JM. Unilateral eccentric contraction of the Plantarflexors leads to bilateral alterations in leg dexterity. Frontiers in Physiology. 2016;**7**:582. DOI: 10.3389/fphys.2016.00582

[24] Cano-de-la-Cuerda R, Molero-Sánchez A, Carratalá-Tejada M, Alguacil-Diego IM, Molina-Rueda F, Miangolarra-Page JC, et al. Theories and control models and motor learning: Clinical applications in neurorehabilitation. Neurología. 2015;**30**:32-41. DOI: 10.1016/j.nrl.2011.12.010

[25] Levin MF, Demers M. Motor learning in neurological rehabilitation. Disability and Rehabilitation. 2021;**43**:3445-3453. DOI: 10.1080/09638288.2020.1752317

[26] Maier M, Ballester BR, Verschure PFMJ. Principles of Neurorehabilitation after stroke based on motor learning and brain plasticity mechanisms. Frontiers in Systems Neuroscience. 2019;**13**:74. DOI: 10.3389/fnsys.2019.00074

[27] Huang VS, Krakauer JW. Robotic neurorehabilitation: A computational motor learning perspective. Journal of Neuroengineering and Rehabilitation. 2009;**6**:5. DOI: 10.1186/1743-0003-6-5

[28] Krakauer JW, Hadjiosif AM, Xu J, Wong AL, Haith AM. Motor learning. Comprehensive. Physiology. 2019;**9**:613-663. DOI: 10.1002/cphy.c170043

[29] Perez MA, Lundbye-Jensen J, Nielsen JB. Changes in corticospinal drive to spinal motoneurones

following visuo-motor skill learning in humans. The Journal of Physiology. 2006;**573**:843-855. DOI: 10.1113/jphysiol.2006.105361

[30] Muellbacher W, Ziemann U, Boroojerdi B, Cohen L, Hallett M. Role of the human motor cortex in rapid motor learning. Experimental Brain Research. 2001;**136**:431-438. DOI: 10.1007/s002210000614

[31] Mendez-Balbuena I, Huethe F, Schulte-Mönting J, Leonhart R, Manjarrez E, Kristeva R. Corticomuscular coherence reflects interindividual differences in the state of the corticomuscular network during low-level static and dynamic forces. Cerebral Cortex. 2012;**22**:628-638. DOI: 10.1093/cercor/bhr147

[32] Patino L, Omlor W, Chakarov V, Hepp-Reymond MC, Kristeva R. Absence of gamma-range corticomuscular coherence during dynamic force in a deafferented patient. Journal of Neurophysiology. 2008;**99**:1906-1916. DOI: 10.1152/jn.00390.2007

[33] Cohen RA, Marsiske MM, Smith GE. Neuropsychology of aging. Handbook of Clinical Neurology. 2019;**167**:149-180. DOI: 10.1016/B978-0-12-804766-8.00010-8

[34] Harada CN, Natelson Love MC, Triebel KL. Normal cognitive aging. Clinics in Geriatric Medicine. 2013;**29**:737-752. DOI: 10.1016/j.cger.2013.07.002

[35] Byrne C, Faure C, Keene DJ, Lamb SE. Ageing, muscle power and physical function: A systematic review and implications for pragmatic training interventions. Sports Medicine. 2016;**46**:1311-1332. DOI: 10.1007/s40279-016-0489-x

[36] Austad SN, Wood MA, Villeda SA, Voss JL, Sahay A, Albert M. Innovative approaches in cognitive aging. Neurobiology of Aging. 2019;**83**:150-154. DOI: 10.1016/j.neurobiolaging.2019.04.013

[37] Blinkouskaya Y, Caçoilo A, Gollamudi T, Jalalian S, Weickenmeier J. Brain aging mechanisms with mechanical manifestations. Mechanism of Ageing and Development. 2021;**200**:111575. DOI: 10.1016/j.mad.2021.111575

[38] Damoiseaux JS. Effects of aging on functional and structural brain connectivity. NeuroImage. 2017;**160**:32-40. DOI: 10.1016/j.neuroimage.2017.01.077

[39] Pascarella A, Manzo L, Ferlazzo E. Modern neurophysiological techniques indexing normal or abnormal brain aging. Seizure: European. Journal of Epilepsy. 2024;**S1059-1311**(24):00194-8. DOI: 10.1016/j.seizure.2024.07.001

[40] Anderson AJ, Perone S. Developmental change in the resting state electroencephalogram: Insights into cognition and the brain. Brain and Cognition. 2018;**126**:40-52. DOI: 10.1016/j.bandc.2018.08.001

[41] Ferreira LK, Busatto GF. Resting-state functional connectivity in normal brain aging. Neuroscience & Biobehavioral Reviews. 2013;**37**:384-400. DOI: 10.1016/j.neubiorev.2013.01.017

[42] Fan JC, Cheung RT, Chu LW, Fung PCW, Chang CQ, Sik HH, et al. Age-related changes of EEG and its source in resting state. In: 2014 19th International Conference on Digital Signal Processing; 20-23 August 2014. Hong Kong: IEEE; 2014. pp. 797-800. DOI: 10.1109/ICDSP.2014.6900774

[43] Ho MC, Chou CY, Huang CF, Lin YT, Shih CS, Han SY, et al. Age-related

changes of task-specific brain activity in normal aging. Neuroscience Letters. 2012;**507**:78-83. DOI: 10.1016/j.neulet.2011.11.057

[44] Kamp D, Krause V, Butz M, Schnitzler A, Pollok B. Changes of cortico-muscular coherence: An early marker of healthy aging? Age. 2013;**35**:49-58. DOI: 10.1007/s11357-011-9329-y

[45] Johnson AN, Shinohara M. Corticomuscular coherence with and without additional task in the elderly. Journal of Applied Physiology. 2012;**112**:970-981. DOI: 10.1152/japplphysiol.01079.2011

[46] Noble JW, Eng JJ, Kokotilo KJ, Boyd LA. Aging effects on the control of grip force magnitude: An fMRI study. Experimental Gerontology. 2011;**46**:453-461. DOI: 10.1016/j.exger.2011.01.004

[47] Yoshida T, Masani K, Zabjek K, Chen R, Popovic MR. Dynamic cortical participation during bilateral, cyclical ankle movements: Effects of aging. Scientific Reports. 2017;**7**:44658. DOI: 10.1038/srep44658

[48] Bayram MB, Siemionow V, Yue GH. Weakening of corticomuscular signal coupling during voluntary motor action in aging. Journal of Gerontology. Series A, Biological Sciences and Medical Sciences. 2015;**70**:1037-1043. DOI: 10.1093/gerona/glv014

[49] Graziadio S, Basu A, Tomasevic L, Zappasodi F, Tecchio F, Eyre JA. Developmental tuning and decay in senescence of oscillations linking the corticospinal system. Journal of Neuroscience. 2010;**30**:3663-3674. DOI: 10.1523/JNEUROSCI.5621-09.2010

[50] Barthels D, Das H. Current advances in ischemic stroke research and therapies. Biochimica et Biophysia Acta: Molecular Basis of Disease. 2020;**1866**:165260. DOI: 10.1016/j.bbadis.2018.09.012

[51] Arsava EM, Ballabio E, Benner T, Cole JW, Delgado-Martinez MP, Dichgans M, et al. The causative classification of stroke system: An international reliability and optimization study. Neurology. 2010;**75**:1277-1284. DOI: 10.1212/WNL.0b013e3181f612ce

[52] Malik AN, Tariq H, Afridi A, Rathore FA. Technological advancements in stroke rehabilitation. Journal of Pakistan Medical Association. 2022;**72**:1672-1674. DOI: 10.47391/JPMA.22-90

[53] Gittler M, Davis AM. Guidelines for adult stroke rehabilitation and recovery. Journal of the American Medical Association. 2018;**319**:820-821. DOI: 10.1001/jama.2017.22036

[54] Mead GE, Sposato LA, Sampaio Silva G, Yperzeele L, Wu S, Kutlubaev M, et al. A systematic review and synthesis of global stroke guidelines on behalf of the world stroke organization. International Journal of Stroke. 2023;**18**:499-531. DOI: 10.1177/17474930231156753

[55] Ding Q, Chen J, Zhang S, Chen S, Li X, Peng Y, et al. Neurophysiological characterization of stroke recovery: A longitudinal TMS and EEG study. CNS Neuroscience & Therapeutics. 2024;**30**:e14471. DOI: 10.1111/cns.14471

[56] Vatinno AA, Simpson A, Ramakrishnan V, Bonilha HS, Bonilha L, Seo NJ. The prognostic utility of electroencephalography in stroke recovery: A systematic review and meta-analysis. Neurorehabilitation and Neural Repair. 2022;**36**:255-268. DOI: 10.1177/15459683221078294

[57] Keser Z, Buchl SC, Seven NA, Markota M, Clark HM, Jones DT, et al. Electroencephalogram (EEG) with or without transcranial magnetic stimulation (TMS) as biomarkers for post-stroke recovery: A narrative review. Frontiers in Neurology. 2022;**13**:827866. DOI: 10.3389/fneur.2022.827866

[58] Zheng Y, Peng Y, Xu G, Li L, Wang J. Using Corticomuscular coherence to reflect function recovery of paretic upper limb after stroke: A case study. Frontiers in Neurology. 2018;**8**:728. DOI: 10.3389/fneur.2017.00728

[59] Larsen LH, Zibrandtsen IC, Wienecke T, Kjaer TW, Christensen MS, Nielsen JB, et al. Corticomuscular coherence in the acute and subacute phase after stroke. Clinical Neurophysiology. 2017;**128**:2217-2226. DOI: 10.1016/j.clinph.2017.08.033

[60] Aikio R, Laaksonen K, Sairanen V, Parkkonen E, Abou Elseoud A, Kujala J, et al. CMC is more than a measure of corticospinal tract integrity in acute stroke patients. Neuroimage: Clinical. 2021;**32**:102818. DOI: 10.1016/j.nicl.2021.102818

[61] Krauth R, Schwertner J, Vogt S, Lindquist S, Sailer M, Sickert A, et al. Cortico-muscular coherence is reduced acutely post-stroke and increases bilaterally during motor recovery: A pilot study. Frontiers in Neurology. 2019;**10**:126. DOI: 10.3389/fneur.2019.00126

[62] von Carlowitz-Ghori K, Bayraktaroglu Z, Hohlefeld FU, Losch F, Curio G, Nikulin VV. Corticomuscular coherence in acute and chronic stroke. Clinical Neurophysiology. 2014;**125**:1182-1191. DOI: 10.1016/j.clinph.2013.11.006

[63] Nelles G, Spiekermann G, Jueptner M, Leonhardt G, Müller S, Gerhard H, et al. Reorganization of sensory and motor systems in hemiplegic stroke patients. A positron emission tomography study. Stroke. 1999;**30**:1510-1516. DOI: 10.1161/01.str.30.8.1510

[64] Fauvet M, Gasq D, Chalard A, Tisseyre J, Amarantini D. Temporal dynamics of Corticomuscular coherence reflects alteration of the central mechanisms of neural motor control in post-stroke patients. Frontiers in Human Neuroscience. 2021;**15**:682080. DOI: 10.3389/fnhum.2021.682080

[65] Schieber MH, Lang CE, Reilly KT, McNulty P, Sirigu A. Selective activation of human finger muscles after stroke or amputation. Advances in Experimental Medicine and Biology. 2009;**629**:559-575. DOI: 10.1007/978-0-387-77064-2_30

[66] Gao Z, Lv S, Ran X, Wang Y, Xia M, Wang J, et al. Influencing factors of corticomuscular coherence in stroke patients. Frontiers in Human Neuroscience. 2024;**18**:1354332. DOI: 10.3389/fnhum.2024.1354332

[67] Rossiter HE, Eaves C, Davis E, Boudrias MH, Park CH, Farmer S, et al. Changes in the location of cortico-muscular coherence following stroke. Neuroimage: Clinical. 2012;**2**:50-55. DOI: 10.1016/j.nicl.2012.11.002

[68] Bao SC, Leung KW, Tong KY. Cortico-muscular interaction to monitor the effects of neuromuscular electrical stimulation pedaling training in chronic stroke. Computers in Biology and Medicine. 2021;**137**:104801. DOI: 10.1016/j.compbiomed.2021.104801

[69] Simon DK, Tanner CM, Brundin P. Parkinson disease epidemiology, pathology, genetics, and pathophysiology. Clinics in Geriatric Medicine. 2020;**36**:1-12. DOI: 10.1016/j.cger.2019.08.002

[70] Beitz JM. Parkinson's disease: A review. Frontiers in Bioscience (Scholar Edition). 2014;**6**:65-74. DOI: 10.2741/s415

[71] Mazzoni P, Shabbott B, Cortés JC. Motor control abnormalities in Parkinson's disease. Cold Spring Harbor Perspectives in Medicine. 2012;**2**:a009282. DOI: 10.1101/cshperspect.a009282

[72] Rawji V, Latorre A, Sharma N, Rothwell JC, Rocchi L. On the use of TMS to investigate the pathophysiology of neurodegenerative diseases. Frontiers in Neurology. 2020;**11**:584664. DOI: 10.3389/fneur.2020.584664

[73] Maidan I, Zifman N, Hausdorff JM, Giladi N, Levy-Lamdan O, Mirelman A. A multimodal approach using TMS and EEG reveals neurophysiological changes in Parkinson's disease. Parkinsonism & Related Disorders. 2021;**89**:28-33. DOI: 10.1016/j.parkreldis.2021.06.018

[74] Zokaei N, Quinn AJ, Hu MT, Husain M, van Ede F, Nobre AC. Reduced cortico-muscular beta coupling in Parkinson's disease predicts motor impairment. Brain. Communications. 2021;**3**:fcab179. DOI: 10.1093/braincomms/fcab179

[75] Park H, Kim JS, Paek SH, Jeon BS, Lee JY, Chung CK. Cortico-muscular coherence increases with tremor improvement after deep brain stimulation in Parkinson's disease. Neuroreport. 2009;**20**:1444-1449. DOI: 10.1097/WNR.0b013e328331a51a

[76] Yokoyama H, Yoshida T, Zabjek K, Chen R, Masani K. Defective corticomuscular connectivity during walking in patients with Parkinson's disease. Journal of Neurophysiology. 2020;**124**:1399-1414. DOI: 10.1152/jn.00109.2020

[77] Roeder L, Boonstra TW, Kerr GK. Corticomuscular control of walking in older people and people with Parkinson's disease. Scientific Reports. 2020;**10**:2980. DOI: 10.1038/s41598-020-59810-w

[78] Guillaud E, Seyres P, Barrière G, Jecko V, Bertrand SS, Cazalets JR. Locomotion and dynamic posture: Neuro-evolutionary basis of bipedal gait. Neurophysiology Clinique. 2020;**50**:467-477. DOI: 10.1016/j.neucli.2020.10.012

[79] Biotteau M, Albaret JM, Chaix Y. Developmental coordination disorder. Handbook of Clinical Neurology. 2020;**174**:3-20. DOI: 10.1016/B978-0-444-64148-9.00001-6

[80] Biotteau M, Danna J, Baudou É, Puyjarinet F, Velay JL, Albaret JM, et al. Developmental coordination disorder and dysgraphia: Signs and symptoms, diagnosis, and rehabilitation. Neuropsychiatric Disease and Treatment. 2019;**15**:1873-1885. DOI: 10.2147/NDT.S120514

[81] Emanuele M, Polletta G, Marini M, Fadiga L. Developmental coordination disorder: State of the art and future directions from a neurophysiological perspective. Children (Basel). 2022;**9**:945. DOI: 10.3390/children9070945

[82] Hyde C, Fuelscher I, Williams J, Lum JAG, He J, Barhoun P, et al. Corticospinal excitability during motor imagery is reduced in young adults with developmental coordination disorder. Research in Developmental Disabilities. 2018;**72**:214-224. DOI: 10.1016/j.ridd.2017.11.009

[83] Ruddock S, Piek J, Sugden D, Morris S, Hyde C, Caeyenberghs K, et al. Coupling online control and inhibitory systems in children with DevelopmentalCoordination disorder:

Goal-directed reaching. Research in Developmental Disabilities. 2015;**36C**:244-255. DOI: 10.1016/j.ridd.2014.10.013

[84] Parr JVV, Hodson-Tole E, Wood G. Short report presenting preliminary evidence of impaired corticomuscular coherence in an individual with developmental coordination disorder. Research in Developmental Disabilities. 2022;**131**:104355. DOI: 10.1016/j.ridd.2022.104355

Chapter 7

Artificial Intelligence Methods for Recognition of Neuromuscular Diseases

Kamala Oghuz

Abstract

The presented chapter examines using artificial neural networks as a processing tool in medical research. Normal and pathological muscle signals obtained by the electromyography method were selected for study. The main research directions are the recognition of pathological changes in stimulated electromyography through neural networks, the use of artificial intelligence methods in the diagnosis of diseases through electromyographic signals, the decision in the diagnosis of myographic diseases using the modular architecture of the neural network, applying different optimization methods in calculating the error of the neural network for the diagnosis of neuromuscular diseases, using neural networks in the comparative analysis of optimization methods of electromyographic signal classifiers, and classifying electromyographic signals based on a sequential machine learning model using deep learning methods.

Keywords: artificial neural networks, electromyography, diagnostics, NeuroPro, sequential machine learning model, network error, modular architecture, optimization methods

1. Introduction

The application of neural network technologies is aimed at the analysis of information flows, as in a living organism. In a sense, this is the development of computer analysis methods that work on the principle of neural networks (NNs) that make up a living organism. In such an approach, neural technologies are a slightly expanded group of technical means and mathematical methods of information flows, the application of which allows for obtaining the desired results.

Although there are many approaches to explaining neural networks, they all have a common feature. So, they are all very much connected and consist of the same type of elements—neurons, as in the human brain.

The application of neural networks in medical and biological research is multifaceted [1]:

- processing of medical images in order to increase their diagnostic informativeness;
- monitoring of the patient's condition;

- intellectual support to the doctor in diagnostic solutions;
- analysis of treatment effectiveness;
- reducing or compensating the impact of random noise on the measurement accuracy of the recording device, etc.

The versatility of the mentioned fields of application enables the wide application of this technology in the processing of medical data. Based on the results of literature research, it can be noted that today the application of artificial neural networks (ANNs) covers almost all fields of medical and biological research.

Neural network technologies open wide opportunities in medical-biological data processing.

In the material [2], a neural network is used for the diagnosis and prediction of peritonitis based on hemostasis parameters. Here, the input parameters of the network corresponding to 50 normal and 50 pathological conditions are taken. For both layers of the network, the sigmoid was chosen as the activation function (the nonlinear gain property of the neuron), and the sensitivity and specificity were calculated. Outputs (norm and pathology) in the established network are shown in the form of a code consisting of four 0 s and 1 s. It should be noted that the number of such examples is quite large.

There are almost no materials on the application of neural networks in electromyography (EMG). Stimulated electromyography is also measured at the level of numbers.

Boginich and others proposed to realize the study of the dynamics of changes in the position of transverse striated muscles in the lower limbs by recording surface potentials with a neural network [3]. They used an image-transformed Hamming network and multilayer perceptron (MCP) for their research. The range of values varies from −1000 to 1000. The network is built in the Generative Adversarial Networks (GANs) neural network package and consists of one hidden and one output layer. The discretization step was chosen to be 0.01. The working principle of the network is based on the determination of the threshold price. If the examined person's condition exceeds the set threshold value, it is considered normal, otherwise, it is considered pathological.

Neural networks are nonlinear systems that allow better classification of data than the linear methods usually applied. Their addition to medical diagnostics increases the specificity of the method without reducing the sensitivity.

2. Recognition of pathological changes in stimulated electromyography using neural networks

The realization of the study was carried out in the NeuroPro0.25 network emulator. NeuroPro0.25 is a beta version of a free software product designed for working with neural networks.

Let us look at the issues of application of neural networks in the processing and analysis of parameters obtained in stimulated electromyography. Electromyographic parameters of patients with normal muscle system conditions and muscle syndromes —carpal tunnel syndrome, cubital tunnel syndrome, and demyelinated polyneuropathy were taken up for the study.

Myograms of patients in the age range of 45–55 years were used for research purposes.

It should be noted that, depending on the type of research in stimulated EMG, measurement results can be taken from several parts. Registration results are taken from a minimum of 16 points in the registration with the viewed device. However, depending on the severity of the pathology, the number of registration points can be increased. The measurement results were taken from the muscle parts through which the nervus medianus (n.medianus) and nervus ulnaris (n.ulnaris) nerves pass [4].

The structural scheme of the network is given in **Figure 1**.

Informative measured parameters were selected as input parameters. The following substitutions have been made here:

- Sensor – S;
- Motor – M;
- Wrist – W;
- Elbow – E;
- Latency – L;
- Amplitude – A;
- Velocity – V.

Depending on the location of the measurements, the selected neural and informative parameters, the input quantities of the network are shown in **Table 1**.

Database input field for preprocessing for network transmission is calculated according to the formula

$$I = (I - a_i)/b_i \qquad (1)$$

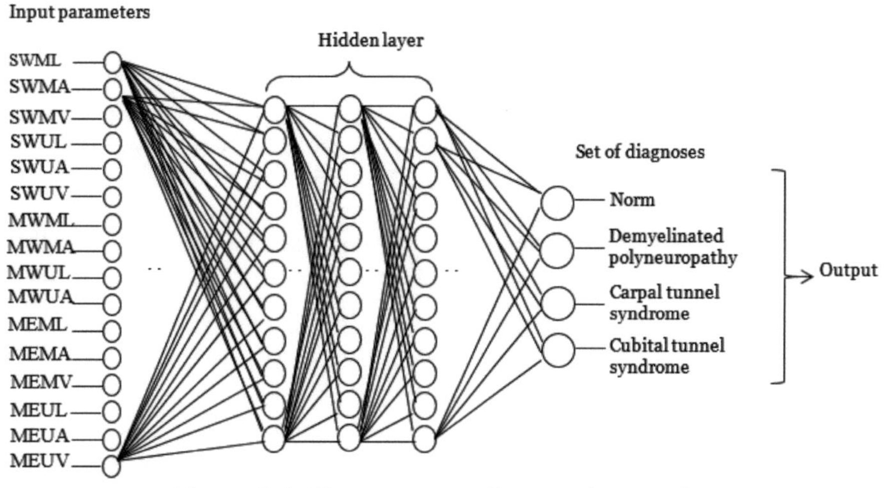

Figure 1.
The structure of a neural network.

Sequence of acquisition of input quantities	Database field (entry syndromes)	Database field (output syndrome)
SensorNCS-wrist-n.medianus-latency	SWML	OUTPUT
SensorNCS-wrist-n.medianus-amplitude	SWMA	
SensorNCS-wrist-n.medianus-velocity	SWMV	
SensorNCS-wrist-n.ulnaris-latency	SWUL	
SensorNCS-wrist-n.ulnaris-amplitude	SWUA	
SensorNCS-wrist-n.ulnaris-velocity	SWUV	
MotorNCS-wrist-n.medianus-latency	MWML	
MotorNCS-wrist-n.medianus-amplitude	MWMA	
MotorNCS-wrist-n.ulnaris-latency	MWUL	
MotorNCS-wrist-n.ulnaris-amplitude	MWUA	
MotorNCS-elbow-n.medianus-latency	MEML	
MotorNCS-elbow-n.medianus-amplitude	MEMA	
MotorNCS-elbow-n.medianus-velocity	MEMV	
MotorNCS-elbow-n.ulnaris-latency	MEUL	
MotorNCS-elbow-n.ulnaris-amplitude	MEUA	
MotorNCS-elbow-n.ulnaris-velocity	MEUV	

Table 1.
The location of measurements, selected neural and informative parameters depending on the input quantities of the network.

where, I is the input quantity; a_i and b_i are calculated coefficients for each entry. Thus, the initial processing of inputs is carried out by the following formulas (weights are automatically determined by the program):

SWML = (SWML-3075)/1075; SWMA = (SWMA-11.8)/4.400001; SWMV = (SWMV-40.75)/14.25; SWUL = (SWUL-1.775)/0.0749; SWUA = (SWUA-11.65)/3.15; SWUV = (SWUV-53.7)/5.1; MWML = (MWML-4575)/2025; MWMA = (MWMA-7.55)/2.45; MWUL = (MWUL-2.5)/0.2; MWUA = (MWUA-9.75)/2.45; MEML = (MEML-8675)/2075; MEMA = (MEMA-6.45)/2.35; MEMV = (MEMV-54.95)/4.35; MEUL = (MEUL-6.725)/0.4749; MEUA = (MEUA-9.25)/2.15; MEUV = (MEUV-53.65)/6.85.

For the network, three hidden layers with 10 neurons each are chosen, and the nonlinearity or transfer function is sigmoidal, the latter being smoothed by the following formula:

$$\boldsymbol{f}(\boldsymbol{X}) = \boldsymbol{X}/(\boldsymbol{c} + |\boldsymbol{X}|) \tag{2}$$

where c is the characteristic of the network and is taken as 0.1.

Using (2), the functional converters in the hidden layers are calculated as follows:

Sigmoid1(A) = A/(0.1 + |A|).

Sigmoid 2(A) = A/(0.1 + |A|).

Sigmoid 3(A) = A/(0.1 + |A|).

The output area of the network OUTPUT consists of four elements and they are:

1. norm;
2. demyelinating polyneuropathy;
3. carpal tunnel syndrome;
4. cubital tunnel syndrome.

After the network is trained, the result of the new parameters entered as an example is shown in **Figure 2**.

As can be seen from the figure, the new measurement results correspond to the "1" state of the output, that is, the normal state.

As mentioned, the Neural network system also allows optimization of the number of input parameters. Thus, in medical research, obtaining multiple input parameters is not desirable from the point of view of having a painful effect and prolonging the research time.

The determination of the degree of importance for the input parameters in the considered network is shown in **Figure 3**.

№	OUTPUT	Network Forecast	Error
1	1	0,8340689	0,1659311
2	2	2,289162	-0,2891622
3	3	2,765857	0,2341425
4	4	3,99793	0,00206995
5		0,8126549	

Figure 2.
Input to the network after training the result of new measurements.

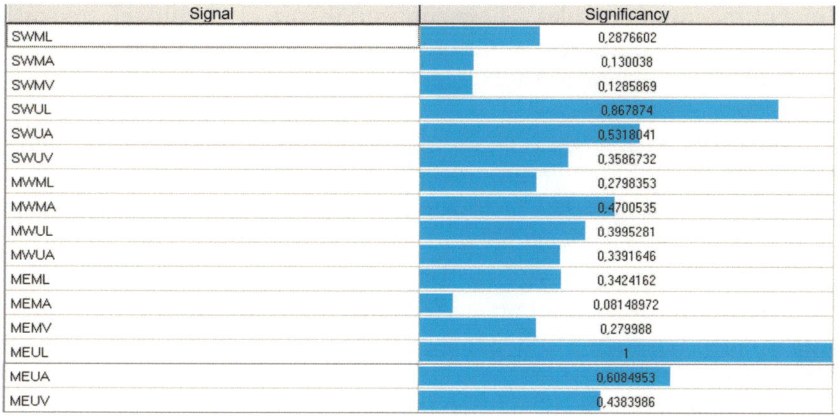

Figure 3.
Signifcance of input parameters.

It can be clearly seen from **Figure 3** that despite including 16 measurement results as input parameters, only the values obtained from MEUL, SWUL, SWUA, and MEUA points are selected more according to the degree of significance.

It should be noted that the NeuroPro software overlay performs the training automatically.

3. Using the modular architecture of the neural network to make decisions on the diagnosis of myographic diseases

Multipurpose artificial neural networks (ANNs) have a monological structure. Such networks work well with small output data, but as the input data increase, the complexity of the network increases and its capacity decreases [5]. To overcome this problem, researchers choose the concept of modularity, and in this case, the problem lies in the choice of modules and structures.

In Mui et al. [6], locally connected adaptive modular NNs are presented. This model works with backpropagation (BP) learning and the structural layers are arranged in a winner-take-all fashion.

The article mentioned in Bellotti et al. [7] presents a modular neural network with a self-organizing map and a multilayer perceptron (MLP) for cosmic radiation experiments.

Research methodology. Due to the proposed modular architecture, the number of weight connections is less compared to a fully connected multilayer perceptron. The module is designed to combine two different generalization approaches known from network connections and logical neural networks, which increases the generalization capabilities of the network.

The architecture presented here is particularly useful for solving problems with large numbers of input attributes. If the input size is small, the network can be trained very quickly, but the performance of the BP algorithm decreases for large input gaps. In many cases, it is important for a number of parameters that lead to an approach to an acceptable minimum. This makes it an often useful solution, especially when identifying large input gaps. Much research is being done to overcome these problems, and such ideas include modularity as a key concept.

The proposed network system consists of a layer of input modules and an additional decision-making module. All subnets are MLP. Each input variable is connected to only one of the input modules. These connections are randomly selected and the outputs of all input modules are connected to the decision-making network.

The following parameters are assumed: the size of the input vector is l, and the number of classes is k.

One of the design challenges is choosing the number of inputs (n) for each module in the first layer; this solution defines the number of input modules $m = \lceil 1/n \rceil$ (presumably $l = m^*n$, if not, then spare inputs are connected to permanent inputs or one of them can be resized). Each network of the first level has $\lceil \boldsymbol{log_2 k} \rceil$ outputs. This is the number required to represent all classes in binary code. The decision network has $\boldsymbol{m} \lceil \boldsymbol{log_2 k} \rceil$ inputs, and the number of outputs is k neurons per class. The number of weights is much less than a fully connected monolithic MLP with the same number of hidden neurons.

In the first stage, all the auxiliary networks in the input layer are trained, and the test set for each subnet is selected from the initial test set. All the input modules can easily be developed in parallel because they all depend on each other.

In the second stage, the decision-making system is taught. The training set for the decision module is built on the output of the input layer along with the original class number. To compute the set, each input pattern is applied to the input layer, the resulting vector together with the desired output class (represented in l-out-of-k encoding) forms the training pair for the decision module.

The original trainer network:

$$\left(x_1^j, x_2^j, \dots, x_i^j; d^j\right), \quad j = 1, 2, \dots, t \tag{3}$$

where $x_i^j \in R$ – the ith component of the jth input vector; d^j – class number; and t – the number of trained samples.

The MLPi module (i-th layer in module) is connected:

$$x_{i \cdot n+1}, x_{i \cdot n+2}, \dots, x_{(i+1) \cdot n} \tag{4}$$

A trainer network of the MLPi network:

$$\left(x_{i \cdot n+1}^j, x_{i \cdot n+2}^j, \dots, x_{(i+1) \cdot n}^j; d_{BIN}^j\right), j = 1, 2, \dots, t \tag{5}$$

here, d_{BIN}^j —is the binary coded number of the class.

Representation of implementations with input layer

$$\Phi : R^{n*m} \to R^{m*\lceil log_2 k \rceil} \tag{6}$$

A trainer network of a decision-making network

$$\Phi\left(x_1^j, x_2^j, \dots, x_i^j; d_{BIN}^j\right); j = 1, 2, \dots, t \tag{7}$$

Description of the network of solutions

$$\Psi : R^{m*\lceil log_2 k \rceil} \to R^k \tag{8}$$

Calculation of output. A description of the entire network

$$\Phi o \Psi : R^l \to R^k \tag{9}$$

Here, o - Φ **and** Ψ denote the composition of images. Thus, for every element of R^l, there is one and only one element of R^k.

For a given input signal $(a_1, a_2, \dots, a_l)$, the response r is determined by the following function

$$r = \Psi(\Phi(a_1, a_2, \dots, a_l)). \tag{10}$$

The k-dimensional output of the decision module is used to determine the class number for that input. In experiments, the output neuron with the highest response is selected as the computed class. The differences between the winning neuron and the runner-up can be taken as a measure of accuracy.

The ability to generalize is a key feature of neural networks. In this way, neural networks can process inputs that are not learned but are similar to those observed in the training phase. Generalization can generally be viewed as a method of drawing from a set of examples. Such reasoning is not correct in a logical context, but can be observed in human behavior.

This architecture combines two generalization methods. One way to generalize is to build in the MLP. Each of the networks has the ability to generalize in its input space. This type of generalization is common to relational systems. Another method of generalization is related to the architecture of the proposed network. This method of generalization is consistent according to the similarity of uniformity of input parameters and is used in logical neural networks.

The general scheme of the proposed structure of the modular network is shown in **Figure 4**.

Let us consider such a structure using the example of diagnosis of myographic diseases.

Values of amplitudes, speed, and delay from 16 points of upper limb muscles were selected as input parameters. Depending on the values of the repeated measurements and taking into account the individuality of the subjects, it is important to choose the interval values of the input parameters. The main problem in this approach is step selection.

Numerous sources suggest choosing a constant step, but this is not very effective in real work. Depending on the choice of network method, there are several stepwise selection algorithms. More successful, although simple to implement, is an algorithm whose idea is to increase the step as the error decreases and decrease as it increases [8].

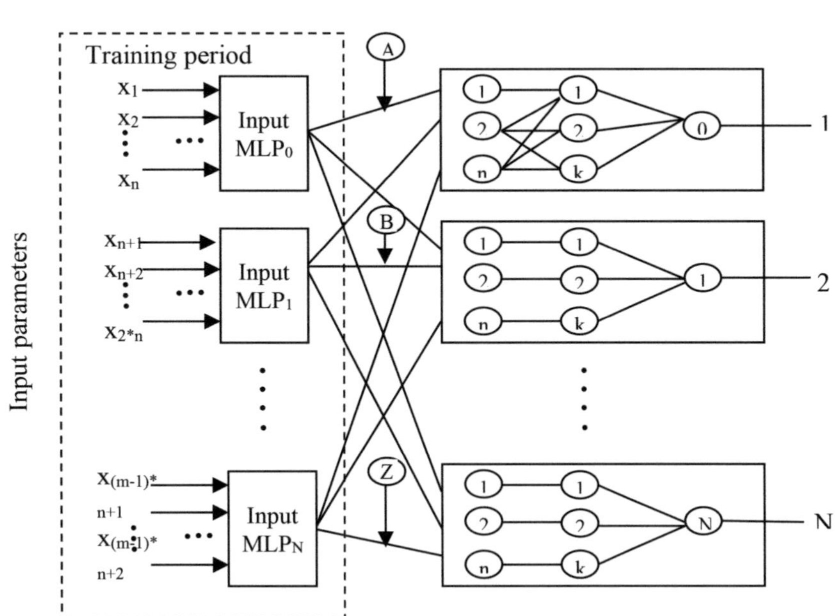

Figure 4.
General scheme of the modular network structure.

The advantage of the modular structure is that each module concentrates its resources on the recognition of only one pathology, which reduces the probability of an incorrect result error for the whole system, but its individual modules do not have information about all types of pathologies. Therefore, a multilayer perceptron was used for the experiment [9].

A generalized structure of a multilayer perceptron can be seen in **Table 2**.

X1-X16 in the table – data entered with one value - [·]; Y - network output (types of studied myographic diseases are coded here): 1 - norm; 2 - carpal tunnel syndrome; 3 - cubital tunnel syndrome; and 4 - demyelinating polyneuropathy.

The proposed version of the modular structure of the training network can be presented in **Table 3**.

In the table [⋯] - set of values for each module - input values, X1-X16 - input modules, Z - MLP output: L (latency (delay)), A (amplitude), and V (velocity).

The decision-making network of the modular structure is presented in **Table 4**.

To evaluate the effectiveness of the diagnostic system, the recommended criteria for the sensitivity and specificity of the network for a certain pathology were used (**Table 5**).

X1	X2	…	X16	Y
[·]	[·]	…	[·]	1
[·]	[·]	…	[·]	2
[·]	[·]	…	[·]	3
[·]	[·]	…	[·]	4

Table 2.
Generalized structure of a multilayer perceptron.

X1	X2	…	X16	Z
[⋯]	[⋯]	…	[⋯]	L
[⋯]	[⋯]	…	[⋯]	A
[⋯]	[⋯]	…	[⋯]	V

Table 3.
Trainer network of modular structure.

Modules			Y
L	A	V	
[⋯]	[⋯]	[⋯]	1
[⋯]	[⋯]	[⋯]	2
[⋯]	[⋯]	[⋯]	3
[⋯]	[⋯]	[⋯]	4

In the table: L, A, V - decision network modules; Y - network output: 1 - norm; 2 - carpal tunnel syndrome; 3 - cubital tunnel syndrome; and 4 - demyelinating polyneuropathy.

Table 4.
Decision-making network.

Output	Sensitivity	Specificity
A multilayer perceptron		
Y1	95,67	98,45
Y2	75,80	95,64
Y3	90,89	99,42
Y4	82,40	98,30
Average value	86,19	97,95
Modular structure		
Y1	99,78	100
Y2	100	100
Y3	95,77	99,45
Y4	68,10	98,99
Average value	90,91	99,61

Table 5.
Using the proposed structures of neural networks, the results of the experiment.

The results of the experiment show that the modular structure of the neural network is more efficient because the average value of the sensitivity criterion for the structure of the multilayer perceptron was 86.19, and 97.95 for the specificity. At the same time, these indicators for modular structure were 90.91 for sensitivity and 99.61 for specificity, respectively.

The generalization advantages for high-dimensional input vectors and the ease of parallel learning at the input level due to the independence of the modules underlie the possibility of using the proposed structure in the diagnosis of diseases in myography.

4. Application of various optimization methods in calculating the error of the neural network for the diagnosis of neuromuscular diseases

An artificial neural network (ANN) is a system of simple processors that are connected and interconnected. Perceptron is one of the first models of neural networks. A perceptron is capable of learning and is based on statistics. Image information is distributed by weighting coefficients (similar to the coefficients of a system of equations) that together describe certain fragments of the image.

There are many approaches for processing EMG signals using these algorithms in information sources. In Akhila Devi and Priyadharsini [10], different types of learning methods were used to classify EMG signals. The model automatically classifies EMG signals as normal, myopathic, and neuropathic. Various feature extraction techniques, such as discrete wavelet transform (DWT) and autoregressive modeling (AR), are used to extract useful information from EMG. An adaptive neuro-fuzzy inference system (ANFIS) with hybrid learning algorithm, support vector machine (SVM), and fuzzy support vector machine (FSVM) enables the classification of EMG signals by comparing accuracy.

In Kehri et al. [11], classification of neuromuscular diseases from electromyography (EMG) signals is proposed, based on a combination of different methods and types of classifiers for object extraction. The combination of wavelet transform (WT) and support vector machine (SVM) improves classification accuracy compared to other combinations.

Researchers like Sailesh Conjeti and Bijay Kumar Rout in [12] monitored the electrophysiological activity of muscles using biofeedback obtained from electromyographic signals collected at the corresponding points of innervation. A comprehensive method for the detection of neuromuscular diseases in a subject and a continuous therapeutic assessment strategy using a rehabilitation assessment matrix are proposed. The decision-making tool was developed using a wide range of physiologic data, including varying degrees of myopathy and neuropathy, from baseline to acute stages. Statistical, spectral, and cepstral features extracted from EMG were used to develop a cascade correlation neural network classifier for disease assessment. The diagnostic yield of the classifier is 91.2% accuracy, 85.3% specificity, and 91.35% sensitivity. The strategy has also been expanded to include isotonic contractions in addition to static isometric contractions. This comprehensive strategy is offered to help physicians plan treatment procedures to maximize the therapeutic value of the rehabilitation process.

Intelligence computing and machine learning techniques such as artificial neural networks (ANNs) serve as powerful tools for analyzing EMG signals and creating optimal myoelectric control schemes for prostheses. The study by Ludermir et al. [13] analyzes the performance of four different neural network structures (forward, recurrent, backpropagation, and self-organizing map) tasked with classifying walking speed when using EMG inputs from 14 different leg muscles. Experiments on the dataset show that self-organizing neural network maps can classify walking speed with over 99% accuracy.

Support vector machine (SVM) is a machine learning technique widely used by many biomedical signal classification applications. In the study by Subasi [14], a novel particle mass optimization (PSO)-SVM model of hybridized particle mass optimization (PSO) and SVM was proposed to improve the classification accuracy of EMG signals.

This optimization mechanism involves adjusting the kernel parameters in the SVM training procedure, which significantly affects the classification accuracy. Experiments were performed based on the EMG signal for classification as normal, neurogenic, or myopathic. The obtained results clearly confirm the superiority of the SVM method over conventional machine learning methods and show that the proposed PSO-SVM classification system provides additional significant improvements in terms of classification accuracy.

In Ludermir et al. [13], a methodology for the global optimization of a neural network is presented. The goal is to simultaneously optimize a multilevel perceptron weight and architecture (MLP) to produce a highly connected, highly classified topo for any given dataset. This approach combines the advantages of a simulation model and a backpropagation learning algorithm to create an automated network design process with a high classification rate and low complexity. Experimental results obtained with four classification problems and one prediction problem performed better than those obtained with the most commonly used optimization methods.

The article mentioned in Nurhazimah et al. [15] provides an overview of the numerous methods available for movement pattern recognition of both isotonic and isometric EMG signals. Various signal analysis methods are compared, showing their applicability in real-time settings. This is especially interesting for researchers who want to choose the most appropriate methodology for classifying movements for different types of contractions. The main function of this study for feature extraction will be the probability density function (PDF) of EMG signals. After a brief description of different methods of preprocessing, feature extraction, and classification of EMG signals, we will compare them in terms of performance.

4.1 A method of calculating the errors of neural networks

It is known that the results of errors are the most important and most accessible indicators of such systems. Absolute and relative errors (errors), which are the most common and at the same time easy to calculate, are calculated by the following formulas [16]:

Absolute error:

$$X_A = P_{sh} - P_h, \tag{11}$$

Relative error:

$$X_R = \frac{P_{sh} - P_h}{P_h} \bullet 100 \tag{12}$$

where $\mathbf{P}_{sh}$ is the response (diagnosis) of the network and $\mathbf{P}_h$ is the actual diagnosis (input value).

Electromyographic signals in normal and pathological conditions were selected for the experiment: carpal tunnel syndrome, cubital tunnel syndrome, and demyelinating neuropathy. The data of 16 measurement points were selected for diagnostics as input parameters of the network. Twenty-six normal and 34 pathological signals were used to create the training complex of the network.

OUTPUT network's output consists of four elements:

1 - norm; 2 - polyneuropathy; 3 - carpal tunnel syndrome; and 4 - cubital tunnel syndrome

The computer implementation of the experiment was carried out in the NeuroPro 0.25 software environment, and optimization methods were selected for network

Given	Received	Absolute error	Relative error
1	1.2463	0.2463	24.6313
1	1.2538	0.2538	25.3780
1	1.1084	0.1084	10.8361
1	1.2290	0.2290	22.9043
2	1.7661	−0.2339	−11.6943
2	2.1642	0.1642	8.2084
2	2.2029	0.2029	10.1441
3	2.7355	−0.2645	−8.8180
3	2.7288	−0.2712	−9.0384
4	4.2662	0.2662	6.6550
4	3.8891	−0.1109	−2.7716
4	4.2564	0.2564	6.4100

Table 6.
A part of the prediction result obtained by the "Gradient Descent" optimization method using a multilayer perceptron.

Given	Received	Absolute error	Relative error
1	1.2988	0.2988	29.8753
1	1.2725	0.2725	27.2539
1	1.1259	0.1259	12.5930
1	1.2302	0.2302	23.0237
2	1.7203	−0.2797	−13.9873
2	2.1983	0.1983	9.9146
2	2.2777	0.2777	13.8863
3	2.7718	−0.2282	−7.6082
3	2.7404	−0.2596	−8.6537
4	3.9893	−0.0107	−0.2681
4	3.7240	−0.2760	−6.9007
4	3.9131	−0.0869	−2.1725

Table 7.
A part of the prediction result obtained by the Modified Par Tan optimization method using a multilayer perceptron.

Given	Received	Absolute error	Relative error
1	1.2193	0.2193	21.9344
1	1.2832	0.2832	28.3217
1	1.0870	0.0870	8.7026
1	1.1494	0.1494	14.9437
2	1.7178	−0.2822	−14.1088
2	2.1470	0.1470	7.3521
2	2.8329	0.8329	41.6473
3	2.8329	−0.1671	−5.5685
3	2.7245	−0.2755	−9.1838
4	4.2747	0.2747	6.8685
4	3.9931	−0.0069	−0.1729
4	4.2719	0.2719	6.7966

Table 8.
A part of prediction result obtained by "Conjugate gradient" optimization method using multilayer perceptron.

training: gradient descent, modified Par Tan, conjugate gradients, and Broyden-Fletcher-Goldfarb-Shanno (BFGS) [17].

Fragments of the results of the first experiment and error calculation are given in **Tables 6–9**.

The number of error values per selected interval was used to compare the optimization methods. Five intervals are selected for absolute errors. The value of the

Given	Received	Absolute error	Relative error
1	1.2903	0.2903	29.0290
1	1.2729	0.2729	27.2865
1	1.1298	0.1298	12.9763
1	1.2034	0.2034	20.3440
2	1.7179	−0.2821	−14.1065
2	2.1506	0.1506	7.5296
2	2.2543	0.2543	12.7168
3	2.7295	−0.2705	−9.0155
3	2.7724	−0.2276	−7.5863
4	4.0351	0.0351	0.8785
4	4.0744	0.0744	1.8596
4	4.0764	0.0764	1.9106

Table 9.
A part of the prediction result obtained by the "BFGS" optimization method using multilayer perceptron.

Ordinal number of the experiment	The number of absolute errors in the corresponding interval				
	< 0.05	0.05–0.09	0.1–0.19	0.2–0.29	> 0.3
1	0	0	3	9	0
2	0	2	2	8	0
3	1	1	3	7	0
4	1	2	2	7	0

Table 10.
Comparison of absolute errors.

Ordinal number of the experiment	Number of relative errors in the corresponding interval				
	< 1	1–9	10–19	20–29	> 30
1	0	6	3	3	0
2	1	5	3	3	0
3	1	6	2	2	1
4	1	5	3	3	0

Table 11.
Comparison of relative errors.

intervals and the number of absolute errors falling into the corresponding interval are shown in **Table 10**.

Five intervals were chosen to compare optimization methods using relative errors [18]. The values of the intervals and the number of relative errors falling into the respective intervals are given in **Table 11**.

Comparison of results was made considering large error values and small number of errors. Thus, the results of Experiments 1 and 2 give a large number of errors with large values (**Table 10**). Despite the fact that the number of errors in the results of the third and fourth experiments was not much different, the fourth option was chosen considering the small number of errors in the third interval.

Similar considerations can be made for the values of **Table 11**. Here, the values of Experiments 2 and 4 coincide, but in this experiment, the best results are obtained in **Table 10**, so option 4 is chosen.

Comparison of optimization methods using network errors allows us to conclude that the best results for the task are obtained using the BFGS optimization method.

This approach will facilitate the work of researchers in choosing an optimization method when working with neural networks for the problem of diagnosing neuromuscular diseases in terms of network error estimation.

5. Use of neural networks in comparative analysis of optimization methods of classifiers of electromyographic signals

The neural network approach to the diagnosis of human conditions is widely used in electrocardiography, electroencephalography, genetics, cancer treatment, etc. In our opinion, the neural network approach is also very promising in electromyography, and we will justify it with experimental results.

Among all types of problems solved on the basis of previous experience, classification problems form a fairly significant group. For them, the answer is to specify a class—a choice of one of several possible solutions [19].

All stepwise optimization methods consist of two most important parts: choosing a direction and choosing a step in that direction. One-dimensional (1D) optimization techniques provide an efficient way to select the step.

Using the optimal step in multicriteria optimization problems, it is impossible to consider the criteria "one by one"—first the value of one is improved, then the other, and so on. It is necessary to synthesize the generalized (integral) criterion. The simplest option is the sum of all. A little more difficult—addition with weights.

A realistic choice of S for one-dimensional optimization is the direction of the antigradient. At each step, this direction is selected, then a one-dimensional optimization is performed, then the gradient H is calculated again, and so on. This is the steepest descent method, the most primitive of the gradient methods. Sometimes it works well.

$p_k = -f(x_k)$ at each step in the gradient descent method. If $f(x_k) \neq 0$, the condition $(f(x_k), p_k) < 0$ is clearly satisfied. Therefore, the direction of the vector p_k is the direction of decrease of the function $f(x)$, and in the immediate neighborhood of the point x_k, the direction pk provides the fastest decrease of this function. For strongly convex functions, the gradient descent method guarantees that the sequence $\{x_k\}$ converges to the minimum point x of the function $f(x)$. The degree of convergence of the method is linear [20].

In the iterative procedure, the direction of the antigradient was used as the direction of the decrease of the function $f(x)$ in the gradient descent methods: $p_k = -f(x_k)$. However, such a choice of the decreasing direction is not always successful. In particular, for unconditional minimization problems, the direction of the antigradient at the point xk may differ significantly from the direction toward the minimum point x. As a result, the trajectory of approaching the minimum point has a zigzag character. The conjugate gradient method takes a different approach. An iterative process is used.

When implementing the conjugate gradient method, a practical technique is used—at every N step, assuming βm N = 0, m = 1,2, … ., the method is updated. The numbers mN are called restart moments. It is often assumed that the dimensions of the En space are N = n. If N = 1, then we get a special case of the conjugate gradient method—the steepest descent method [21].

The modified Par Tan method also requires an additional parameter map to be stored. It is constructed as follows: two steps are taken from a_0 to h: shortest descent. We get a_1, a_2. Then we get a one-dimensional optimization from a_0 to $a_2 - a_0$ - a_3. After that, a_0 is no longer used. Then we get the fastest descent from a_3 to a_4. Then we get a one-dimensional optimization from a_2 to a_4 - a_2, a_S, and so on. Even a2k 2 k-l is obtained by a one-dimensional optimization in the direction s = a2k-a2k-2 by steepest descent from a single a2k + 1 - a2k–2 (initial step h = 1, increasing immediately). The augmentation procedure obtains the values of a_0, s, h_0 and the minimized function h (a_0), H(a_0 + h_oS)'. In this case, h(a_0) ~ H(a_0 + h_oS)'. The calculation procedure uses the minimized function. According to many observations, the modified Par Tan method performs better than k-partan in learning tasks.

The BFGS method, an iterative numerical optimization method, is named after its researchers: Broyden, Fletcher, Goldfarb, and Shanno. It belongs to a class called quasi-Newtonian methods. Unlike Newtonian methods, the Hessian of a function is not directly calculated in quasi-Newtonian methods, i.e. there is no need to find partial second derivatives. Instead, the Hessian is approximated based on the steps taken so far [22].

The value of the Lipschitz constant (LS) serves as an indicator of sample complexity. LS of sample $\{\boldsymbol{x}^i, \boldsymbol{y}^i\}, \boldsymbol{i} = \mathbf{1}, \ldots \boldsymbol{N}$ is equal to

$$\boldsymbol{L}_{\{x^i, y^i\}} = \max_{i \neq j} \frac{\|\boldsymbol{y}^i - \boldsymbol{y}^j\|}{\|\boldsymbol{x}^i - \boldsymbol{x}^j\|} \tag{13}$$

where, $\boldsymbol{x}^i \ \boldsymbol{R}^n, \boldsymbol{y}^i \ \boldsymbol{R}^m$ are vectors of input signals and required output signals of the neural network. It was shown in Ref. [23] that the LS of the sample affects the learning process and the properties of the trained network, and LS should be minimized during sample preprocessing.

Another feature of neural networks is the indicator of the importance of the p-parameter, which is determined by the following formula when solving the q-example.

$$\chi_p^q = \left| \frac{\partial \boldsymbol{H}_q}{\partial \boldsymbol{w}_p} \left(\boldsymbol{w}_p - \boldsymbol{w}_p^* \right) \right| \tag{14}$$

The importance indicator (14) can be calculated for different objects. It is often calculated for trained network parameters. However, the significance indicator of the form (13) also applies to signals. A network in inverse operation always computes two gradient vectors—the trained network parameters and the gradient of the evaluation function for all network signals. If the importance score is calculated to identify the least important neuron, then the importance score of the output signal of the neuron must be calculated. Similarly, in the task of determining the least significant input signal, it is necessary to calculate the importance of this signal, and not the sum of the importance of the weights of the links to which this signal is applied.

Unlike expert systems that work according to known rules, problem solving based on experience is always fuzzy, that is, it includes elements of uncertainty and doubt. It is very similar to human decision-making, where there is always the possibility of making a mistake, even if it is a very small one. Therefore, in addition to the class of

Experiments	Optimization method	Lipschitz constant value	Number of training periods	Step	Important entries	Test results
1	Descent Gradient	1024	70	0,0492	3	95,5%
2	Modified Par Tan	1008	100	0,0556	4	97,75%
3	Converging gradients	1008	16	0,0423	4	94%
4	BFGS	1024	14	0,1665	2	97,5%

Table 12.
Experimental results.

the tested sample, the network calculates the percentage of confidence in this solution. A very practical conclusion follows from this. By changing the values of the sample parameters in different directions and repeating the tests, you can see what and how much should be changed so that the sample belongs to the required class. This can be invaluable for medical diagnosis and prognosis, for example.

In the diagnosis of electromyographic signals for practice, they were selected in normal and pathology to classify the human condition [24]. Inputs and outputs of the network for expemental part are given in **Table 3** in this material.

Four experiments are conducted and the optimization method is changed in each of them. For each experiment, the optimal number of exercise cycles and step for interval values were selected under constant conditions.

After that, significant entries are obtained (significant entries with 0.5 as the limit value and value greater than the limit value are used to select the significant parameters) and test results. The experimental results are shown in **Table 12**.

By comparing the results of the experiments, it can be seen that the properties of the network depend on the choice of the optimization method and change. For the value of the Lipschitz constant, Experiments 2 and 3 show good results. Experiments 1 and 3 can be selected for the step of sample values. The number of significant entries is more in Experiments 2 and 3. The best test result was demonstrated in Experiments 2 and 4. Obviously, this comparison is relative. The choice of features depends on the requirements of the experiment.

In our example, the second experiment can be considered the best for the created network. The best test result is also recorded in this practice—97.75%.

Thus, comparing the properties of neural networks allows choosing the optimization method with a higher value of the network result.

6. Classification of electromyographic signals based on a sequential machine learning model using deep learning methods

Modern processing methods are used in almost all fields of medicine. Artificial intelligence (AI) methods are successfully used to improve diagnostic results.

In Sangwoo Nam et al. [25], researchers propose a method to classify three types of resting membrane potential signals obtained as images through diagnostic needle electromyography (EMG) using TensorFlow-Slim and Python to implement an AI-based image recognition scheme.

The authors Park and Lee of Ref. [26] present an electromyographic (EMG) pattern recognition method to determine movement commands to control a prosthetic hand by gathering evidence based on artificial intelligence with multiple parameters. Integral absolute value, variance, autoregressive (AR) model coefficients, linear cepstrum coefficients, and adaptive cepstrum vector are extracted as feature parameters from several time segments of EMG signals. Pattern recognition is performed by an evidence gathering procedure using distances measured with reference parameters. The fuzzy mapping function is designed to transform the distances to apply the evidence gathering method. Results are presented that confirm the feasibility of the proposed approach for EMG pattern recognition.

In Mahdi and Mehran [27], six unique hand movements were selected to classify myoelectric signals. The features selected for the EMG signal belong to the time and time-frequency domains. In this paper, we demonstrate the capabilities of an EMG pattern recognition system using ANFIS as a classifier with a real-time learning method.

In Ulysse et al. [28], a new multidomain learning algorithm called ADANN (Adaptive Domain Adversarial Neural Network) is presented, which significantly improves cross-disciplinary classification accuracy by 19.40% on average ($p = 0.00004$) compared to standard learning. Using features generated by ADANN, this work presents the first topological analysis of EMG-based gesture recognition data to characterize information encoded in the deep web using manually generated features. This analysis suggests that manual features and learned features (at earlier levels) attempt to discriminate between all gestures, but do not encode the same information to do so. Later levels tend to adopt an all-versus-all strategy for a particular class, instead of learned traits.

The aim of the paper mentioned in Panyawut et al. [29] is to investigate a deep neural network approach to classify 41 hand and wrist movements based on the surface electromyography (sEMG) signal. The proposed models were trained and evaluated using the public database of the Ninapro project, one of the largest publicly available sEMG databases for advanced myoelectric arm prostheses.

A sequential model is a simplified version of a functional model, the simplest linear end-to-end structural sequence without bifurcation and a linear assembly of several network levels.

In general, all layers in Keras need to know the shape of their inputs to be able to generate their weights. So when such a layer is created, it initially has no weight. When an input is first accessed, it creates its own weights because the shape of the weights depends on the shape of the input. Of course, this also applies to Sequential models [30].

When building a new sequential architecture, it is useful to build layers incrementally with add() and print model summaries frequently. For example, it allows you to track how the Conv2D and MaxPooling2D layer stack downsamples the image feature maps.

Once a consistent model is created, it behaves like a functional API model. This means that each layer has an input and an output attribute. These attributes can be used to do cool things like quickly build a model that gets the output of all intermediate layers in a sequential model.

This work is done on the Kaggle platform using the Python programming language. The model used to get the prediction is based on a sequential machine learning model using deep learning methods.

Electromyographic signals of a healthy patient and three common diseases, such as carpal tunnel syndrome, cubital tunnel syndrome, and polyneuropathy, were selected for the experiment [31]. The total number of signals selected for the experiment was 24,000, and the EMG signals were numbered as 0, 1, 2, and 3, respectively.

In programming, all data are divided into two parts, the first of which is 70% of the entire database, which is selected as input. Thirty percent of the total portion is selected as the test base. An excerpt from the program:

Model code:

```
model = Sequential()
model.add(Dense(8, input_dim = input_dim, activation = 'relu'))
model.add(Dense(10, activation = 'relu'))
model.add(Dense(10, activation = 'relu'))
model.add(Dense(10, activation = 'relu'))
model.add(Dense(4, activation = 'softmax'))
model.compile(loss = 'categorical_crossentropy', optimizer = 'adam', metrics = ['accuracy'])
hist = model.fit(train_x, train_y, epochs = 30)
scores = model.evaluate(test_x, test_y)
print("\n%s: %.2f%%" % (model.metrics_names[1], scores[1]*100))
```

Thirty epochs were selected for this network and the result is shown in **Figure 5**.

```
Epoch 22/30
16794/16794 [==============================] - 1s 65us/step - loss: 0.3960 - acc: 0.8011
Epoch 23/30
16794/16794 [==============================] - 1s 60us/step - loss: 0.3928 - acc: 0.8026
Epoch 24/30
16794/16794 [==============================] - 1s 61us/step - loss: 0.3954 - acc: 0.8018
Epoch 25/30
16794/16794 [==============================] - 1s 59us/step - loss: 0.3865 - acc: 0.8057
Epoch 26/30
16794/16794 [==============================] - 1s 61us/step - loss: 0.3892 - acc: 0.8020
Epoch 27/30
16794/16794 [==============================] - 1s 63us/step - loss: 0.3843 - acc: 0.8058
Epoch 28/30
16794/16794 [==============================] - 1s 64us/step - loss: 0.3896 - acc: 0.8024
Epoch 29/30
16794/16794 [==============================] - 1s 63us/step - loss: 0.3863 - acc: 0.8047
Epoch 30/30
16794/16794 [==============================] - 1s 63us/step - loss: 0.3892 - acc: 0.7992
7198/7198 [==============================] - 0s 55us/step

acc: 81.51%
```

Figure 5.
After 30 epochs, the neural network achieved 81.51% accuracy.

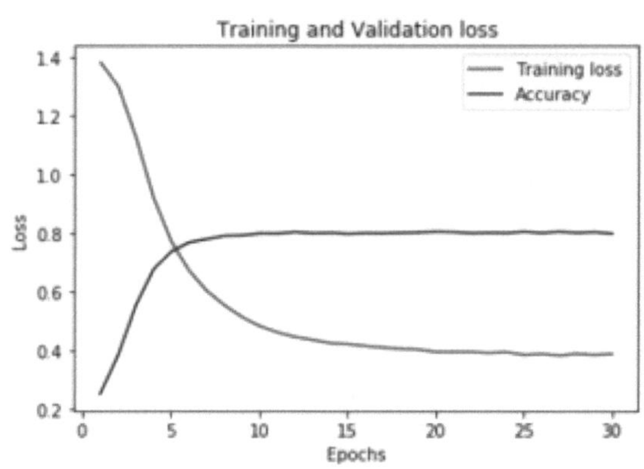

Figure 6.
Learning loss curve.

```
the nn predict 1, and the species to find is 1
the nn predict 0, and the species to find is 0
the nn predict 3, and the species to find is 3
the nn predict 2, and the species to find is 2
the nn predict 0, and the species to find is 0
the nn predict 0, and the species to find is 0
the nn predict 1, and the species to find is 3
the nn predict 2, and the species to find is 2
```

Figure 7.
Network prediction result.

One of the widely used graphs for neural network tuning is the learning loss curve (**Figure 6**). It gives a picture of the learning process and the direction in which the network tends to learn and achieve better results. A loss function is calculated for each data item during one period. Curve fitting to periods gives the loss for each subset of the entire dataset. Another curve that is widely used to understand the progress of neural networks is the accuracy curve. As the training loss decreases, the performance of the neural network will increase. We visualized these two curves together to understand the effect of loss reduction on accuracy improvement.

After training, you can initially make predictions with a small sample extracted from the database. In order to train the neural network, it was necessary to transform the views into vectors. This means that after the prediction, it is necessary to perform an inverse operation to recover the name of the associated species. **Figure 7** shows the network prediction result.

It seems that predicting a small network at the beginning of the selected network works well because the system can clearly predict the input signals. Only one line shows an incorrect prediction, and this is due to very close values of the input signals. This can be fixed by updating the access network.

7. Conclusion

Realization of the neural network in the NeuroPro network emulator was proposed, taking into account the peak amplitude of the signal in the n.medianus and n. ulnaris nerves, the latency period of the motor response, the signal transmission speed, and the distance between the electrodes. As a result of the conducted experiment, the number of input parameters, which are the most important values of the neural network model, was determined. By reducing the number of measurements for the considered case, it allows to shorten the time of the study, and especially, in the needle electromyography method, the patient undergoes less painful procedures.

Neural networks, unlike other expert and diagnostic systems, create multiple combinations of input data to achieve greater approximation to output results. The accuracy of the results of the network was determined based on the training data as a result of the measurement and calculation experiments carried out for diagnostic analysis in the processing of EMG signals.

Computerized neural network diagnostics is the optimal tool in poor information conditions. The proposed structures from multiple neon network models are quite effective from the point of view of prediction, considering the speed of training and high diagnosis accuracy.

Conflict of interest

The author declares no conflict of interest.

Author details

Kamala Oghuz
Baku Higher Oil School, Azerbaijan Technical University, Baku, Azerbaijan

*Address all correspondence to: kamala.pashayeva@bhos.edu.az

References

[1] Evdokimenkov VN. Computer Technologies for Collecting, Processing and Analyzing Data from Biomedical Research. Mai: Tutorial. M; 2005. 436 p. Available from: https://i.twirpx.link/file/1432543/ (in russian)

[2] Sidorova MA, Serzhantova NA, Filippova LA. Diagnosis and prediction of outcomes of peritonitis using a neural network system for studying hemostasis parameters. Medical Technology. 2011; **2**(266):42-47

[3] Boginich AV, Mornev ML, Popov VY. Construction of a high-performance service for intellectual processing of medical information for assessing electromyographic studies of striated muscles. In: Proceedings of the 9th International Conference-Seminar "High-Performance Parallel Computing on Cluster Systems". Vladimir: LLC "Graphics", Triton Studio LLC; 2009. Available from: https://hpc-education.unn.ru/files/conference_hpc/2009/files/proceedings_2009.pdf

[4] Sanadze AG, Kasatkina LF. Clinical Electromyography for a Practicing Neurologist (a Manual for Doctors). Moskov: GEOTAR-Media; 2006. 35 p

[5] Kohonen T, Barna G, Chrisley R. Statistical pattern recognition with neural networks: Benchmarking studies. In: In. Proc. IEEE International Conference on Neural Networks. San Diego: IEEE; 1988. pp. 61-67

[6] Mui L, Agarwal A, Gupta A, Shen-Pei WP. An adaptive modular neural network with application to unconstrained character recognition. International Journal of Pattern Recognition and Artificial Intelligence. 1994;**8**(5):1189-1204

[7] Bellotti R, Castellano M, De Marzo C, Satalino G. Signal/background classification in a cosmic ray space experiment by a modular neural system. In: Proc. of the SPIE - the International Society for Optical Engineering. Vol. 2492. 1995. pp. 1153-1161

[8] Tarkhov DA. Neural Network Models and Algorithms. Directory. Moskov: Radio Engineering; 2014. 352 C. Available from: https://www.gstu.by/sites/default/files/atoms/files/47/f7/tarhanov.pdf (in russian)

[9] Abdullaev NT, Pashaeva KS. Hardware and algorithmic support for an automated device for relaxing muscle tension. Biomedical Radio Electronics. 2021;**23**(2):5-23

[10] Akhila Devi BV, Priyadharsini SS. Diagnosis of neuromuscular disorders using softcomputing techniques. International Journal of Soft Computing and Engineering (IJSCE). 2013;**3**(5): 105-111

[11] Kehri V, Ingle R, Awale R, Oimbe S. Techniques of EMG signal analysis and classification of neuromuscular diseases. Advances in Intelligent Systems Research. 2017;**137**:485-491

[12] Conjeti S, Rout BK. Strategy for electromyography based diagnosis of neuromuscular diseases for assistive rehabilitation. International Journal on Bioinformatics & Biosciences (IJBB). 2013;**3**(3):25-39

[13] Ludermir TB, Yamazaki A, Zanchettin C. An optimization methodology for neural network weights and architectures. IEEE Transactions on Neural Networks. 2006;**17**(6): 1452-1459

[14] Subasi A. Classification of EMG signals using PSO optimized SVM for diagnosis of neuromuscular disorders. Computers in Biology and Medicine. 2013;**43**:576-586

[15] Nurhazimah N et al. A review of classification techniques of EMG signals during isotonic and isometric contractions. Sensors. 2016;**16**:1304-1332

[16] Kulikov LK, Bykova NM, Privalov Yu A, Navtanovich NA, Shabanova OG. Diagnosis of hyperaldosteronism T in patients with adrenal incidentalomas using neural networks. Fundamental Research. 2010;**3**:88-94

[17] Ismayilova KS. Application of various optimization methods when calculating the error of a neural network for diagnosing neuromuscular diseases. Information Technologies, No. 1. 2019; **25**:41-45

[18] Abdullaev NT, Dyshin OA, Khasmamedova GT. Diagnosis of the state of the cardiovascular system based on fractal analysis of RR intervalograms. Biomedical Radioelectronics. 2010;**12**: 25-29

[19] Tsaregorodtsev VG. Optimization of data preprocessing: Lipschitz constant of the training set and properties of trained neural networks. Journal Neurocomputers: Development, Application. 2003;7(7):3-8

[20] Tsaregorodtsev VG. Preprocessing of the training sample, Lipschitz sample constant and properties of trained neural networks. In: Materials of the X Scientific Conference. Seminar "Neuroinformatics and its Applications", Krasnoyarsk. 2002. pp. 146-150

[21] Gorban AN. Training neural networks. In: USSR-USA JV "Para Graph". 1990. 160 p. (English Translation: AMSE Transaction, Scientific Siberian, A, 1993, Vol. 6. Neurocomputing, PP. 1-134). Available from: https://dalab.unn.ru/Gorban/Gorban_Obuchenie_Neironnyh_Setei.pdf (in russian)

[22] BFGS Method or One of the Most Effective Optimization Methods. Example Implementation in Python. Available from: https://habrahabr.ru/post/333356/.

[23] Mirkes EM. Neurocomputer. Draft Standard. 1998. Available from: http://www.gotai.net/documents/doc-nn-006.aspx

[24] Ismailova KS. Application of neural networks in the comparative analysis of methods for optimizing classifiers of electromyographic signals. In: XIII International Scientific Conference Physics and Radioelectronics in Medicine and Ecology, PhREME'2018, Book II. Vladimir: LLC "Graphics"; 2018. pp. 35-39

[25] Nam S, Sohn MK, Kim HA, Kong H-J, Jung I-Y. Development of artificial intelligence to support needle electromyography diagnostic analysis. Healthcare Informatics Research. 2019; **25**(2):400-405. DOI: 10.4258/hir.2019.25.2.131

[26] Park SH, Lee SP. EMG pattern recognition based on artificial intelligence techniques. IEEE Transactions on Rehabilitation Engineering. 1998;**6**(4):400-405. DOI: 10.1109/86.736154

[27] Mahdi K, Mehran J. Real-time intelligent pattern recognition algorithm for surface EMG signals. Biomedical Engineering Online. 2007;**3**(6):45. DOI: 10.1186/1475-925X-6-45

[28] Ulysse CA, Evan C, Phinyomark A, Laviolette F, Gosselin B, Scheme E.

Interpreting deep learning features for myoelectric control: A comparison with handcrafted features. Frontiers in Bioengineering and Biotechnology. 2020;**3**(8):158. DOI: 10.3389/fbioe.2020.00158

[29] Panyawut SI, Chaiyaroj A, Chatchai B, Songphon D, Ronach P, Chusak T, et al. Classification of 41 hand and wrist movements via surface electromyogram using deep neural network. Frontiers in Bioengineering and Biotechnology. 2021;**9**(9):548357. DOI: 10.3389/fbioe.2021.548357

[30] Ways to Build Keras Models. Nerd For Tech; 2021. Available from: https://medium.com/nerd-for-tech/ways-to-build-keras-models-198f6a643944

[31] Abdullaev NT, Pashaeva KS. Classification of electromyographic signals based on a sequential machine learning model using deep learning techniques. In: XV International Scientific Conference Physics and Radioelectronics in Medicine and Ecology – FREM'2022 – Vladimir-Suzdal. LLC "Graphics"; 2022. pp. 263-268

Section 3

Neurological Rehabilitation and Parkinson's Disease

Chapter 8

The Complex and Integrated Rehabilitation Process in Parkinson's Disease

Simona Maria Carmignano

Abstract

Parkinson's disease (PD) gait pattern is conditioned by the typical characteristics of the disease (bradykinesia, rigidity, reduction of amplitude and automaticity of movement). Patients show reduced gait speed and step length, impaired rhythmicity worsened with disease progression. Consequently, gait disturbances influence parkinsonian patients' independence and quality of life. Dopaminergic medications improve only certain gait disturbances such as velocity and step length, while episodic symptoms such as freezing show a variable pharmacological responsiveness. On the other side, dopaminergic medications may negatively influence gait patterns through dyskinesia and motor fluctuations. Rehabilitation is a field addressing responsive care for patients with PD. These approaches include conventional rehabilitation training, auditory and visual cueing training and virtual reality training, treadmill training. In the last 20 years, technological advances have made it possible to develop robotic systems for rehabilitation, which have been added to the traditional methodology.

Keywords: Parkinson's disease, physical exercise, plasticity, technology, rehabilitation

1. Introduction

Parkinson's disease (PD) is a frequent neurodegenerative disease of adulthood, second in prevalence only to Alzheimer's disease. It is associated with a progressive and selective loss of dopaminergic neurons, whose cell bodies are in the substantia nigra pars compacta (SNpc) of the central nervous system (CNS), while the axons and nerve terminals project toward the striatum, the central component of the ganglia of the base and responsible for initiating and controlling the movement [1]. Exactly 200 years have passed since the publication of the famous article "Essay on the Shaking Palsy" by James Parkinson, a young physician who in 1817 described for the first time a disease that, a few years later, would take his name. The description of the motor disorder is so accurate and concise that it is still relevant: "... Involuntary tremulous motion, with lessened muscular power, in parts not in action and even when supported; with a propensity to bend the trunk forwards, and to pass from a walking to a running pace: the senses and intellects being uninjured" [2].

Parkinson's disease (PD) and basal ganglia dysfunction are associated with impaired motor timing, gait disturbances, bradykinesia (slowed movement), hypokinesia (small amplitude movements), resting tremor, rigidity, and postural instability [3]. Postural instability is associated with gait deficits and motor impairment, leading to the onset of alterations and deviations of the column, the occurrence of musculoskeletal pain and a high risk of falling. Falls and its complications together with the fear of falling and cognitive can generate a cascade of events difficult to break, such as isolation and therefore quality of life [4].

The complex and integrated therapeutic approach aims to reduce and contain the progression of the disease to maintain functions for longer and improve the quality of life.

Dopaminergic medications partially improve only velocity and step length, while episodic symptoms such as freezing show a variable and limited pharmacological responsiveness. Therefore, the solution to gait problems needs an understanding of multiple mechanisms that determine this impairment. This acquisition is crucial for the definition of targeted interventions in parkinsonian patients. Motor, sensory, affective, and cognitive deficits are all implicated but gait mechanisms in PD are complex and poorly understood [5]. In addition to pharmacological interventions, rehabilitation is responsive care for patients affected by PD [6].

2. Epidemiology

Parkinson's disease is the most prevalent neurodegenerative disease after Alzheimer's disease and is one of the leading causes of neurological disability in individuals over the age of 60 [7]. The incidence is about 20 affected individuals in a population of 100,000 individuals each year and the prevalence is highly variable worldwide, with estimates ranging from 15/100,000 inhabitants in China, to 150–200/100,000 in Europe and North America. Although the etiology of PD is still unknown, the hypothesis of a multifactorial origin that characterizes this disease and in which both environmental and genetic components interact is now accepted. Over the years, several etiological factors have been proposed: heredity, brain lesions, infections, endogenous neurotoxins, environmental factors, and altered gene expressions [8].

Genetic factors play a key role in the development of PD. On the basis of these data, some experimental models have been developed both *in vivo*, through the use of transgenic animals, and *in vitro* on cell cultures, which have allowed to expand the knowledge on PD.

Studies on the pathogenesis of Parkinson's disease have shown, in animal models, that this disease is determined by the progressive accumulation of abnormal aggregates of α-synuclein. The inflammatory process that determines this phenomenon could be systemic, determining correlations with the gastrointestinal system as well. Moreover, the cellular implications in the pathogenesis process highlight the involvement of mitochondrial and lysosomal abnormalities and alterations in cellular oxidation processes [9].

3. Pathophysiology of Parkinson's disease

Parkinson's is the first case of a neurochemical alteration-related brain disease. The initial research on this aspect, back in the 1950s, indicated that patients' brains, when examined posthumously had little amounts of norepinephrine and serotonin and more essentially dopamine which is the main transmitter secreted by neurons in substantia nigra. In addition the overall circuit organization of basal ganglia was elucidated in the 1980s and early 1990s, with the formulation of the model of "direct" and "indirect" striatal output pathways [10].

In the classical model, the direct pathway would facilitate the desired motor activity, while the indirect pathway would inhibit interfering motor activities [11]. The indirect pathway inhibits the thalamus (indirectly activating the common final pathway) and prevents signals from being sent to the cortex. Normally there is a regulation of these pathways by the dopaminergic neurons of the SN (pars compacta) which excite the D1 receptors (cooperating with the cortex and thus favoring the direct pathway) and inhibit the D2 receptors of the Striatum, limiting the excitatory signal coming from the cortex on them. Such models of the motor circuit are not only simplistic but also help to understand how alterations in dopaminergic afferents affect motor performance [12].

4. Clinical manifestations

Cardinal signs of Parkinson's disease include resting tremor, rigidity, bradykinesia, and postural instability.

The onset symptom is, in 70% of cases, tremor, which is usually unilateral, initially affecting one or the other hand. In a small percentage of cases, the onset may be characterized by motor awkwardness, rigidity, and non-specific complaints.

Tremor in Parkinson's disease has distinctive features. It is a tremor present at rest, with a frequency of 3–5 Hz, which improves with the movement of the affected part. It is asymmetrical at the onset of the disease, aggravated by anxiety, contralateral motor activity and walking; disappears during sleep [13].

The tremor generally affects the hand, leg, or chin; it is rhythmic, reduced by movement, and disappears in sleep.

In the hand, it manifests itself with flexion-extension or adduction-abduction movements of the fingers (such as "counting coins" or "making pills"), rarely affects the head and interferes little with voluntary movements even when it is particularly conspicuous.

Bradykinesia is a scientific term that indicates the slowness of the parkinsonian patient in initiating and continuing a movement until blockage (akinesia). The habitual, automatic, and frequent movements that are observed under normal conditions, such as bringing the hand to the face, bending the arms or crossing the legs, are absent or very reduced in parkinsonian patients [14].

Lack of motor control of speech, called hypokinetic dysarthria, affects about 90% of PD patients. It is characterized by vocalization deficits related to the variation in pitch and intensity during speech.

Dysphagia occurs late in Parkinson's disease and is rarely an early symptom. Patients experience this disorder both in the ingestion of liquids and solid foods. Ii is associated with malnutrition, aspiration pneumonia, and mortality. It can be considered both a motor and a non-motor symptom of PD [15, 16].

The motor language disorder of dysarthria is also characterized by difficulties in lexical access is associated with multiple difficulties such as loss of concentration, inability to create logical connections, tendency to persevere and generalized slowing of thought processes. This leads to progressive social isolation [17, 18].

Stiffness is perceived as resistance during the passive movement of the body segments that is uniform throughout the entire range of movement, qualitatively characterized as plastic rigidity. Unlike what happens in muscle contraction secondary to paralysis (spasticity), the increase in resistance to passive movement is not preceded by an initial free interval and remains constant throughout the range of movement, as occurs when a lead rod is bent or when a rubber strip is stretched (plastic hypertonia, different from spastic hypertonia due to lesions of the pyramidal pathways in which the resistance suddenly gives way under the strain of the examiner). Moreover, when the limb is abandoned, it does not recover the original position but remains motionless in the intermediate position, even if it is uncomfortable or difficult to maintain. It is variable in extent and is present in all muscle groups, both flexor and extensor, but it prevails in muscles that maintain a flexed posture, i.e., in the flexor muscles of the trunk and limbs [19].

Parkinson's disease (PD) gait pattern is conditioned by the typical characteristics of the disease (bradykinesia, rigidity, reduction of amplitude and automaticity of movement). Patients show reduced gait speed and step length, impaired rhythmicity worsened with disease progression. Consequently, gait disturbances influence parkinsonian patients' independence and quality of life. Walking in the advanced stage is characterized by difficulty in starting the walk, which is performed with small strides and swipes, and extreme difficulty in changing direction. Typical are freezing and "festination." Freezing is the inability to start or continue movement in the face of sudden environmental changes, for example, when you are forced to change direction, pass through a door or a narrow space [20]. The pathophysiological mechanisms of this phenomenon are still controversial. One study [21], looking at gait changes immediately preceding the freezing episode, found that this was due to the inability to take steps of adequate length and to maintain rhythm in walking, and increased gait variability. Festination is the tendency to progressively increase the speed of the stride which often leads to falls. Due to its peculiarities, effects on patients' quality of life and possible pathophysiogenetic mechanisms, some authors believe that this symptom should be added to the three "cardinal" motor symptoms (rigidity, tremor, and bradykinesia) for clinical diagnosis. Festination occurs as the patient shifts his or her center of gravity forward, due to involuntary flexion of the trunk. To keep the center of gravity within the support base, safeguard balance and prevent falls, patients increase the speed of walking by taking small, rapid steps until they replace the "run" of walking. The patient pursues his or her center of gravity [22].

In the early stage, the gait of the patient shows step leg shorten, reduced gait speed timing of step swing duration and amplitude of arm swing; besides, is frequent interlimb asymmetry and, also, range of motion of the hip, knee and ankle is reduced with consequent posture modification; complex locomotor task and dual task initially became to be impaired. In the mild to moderate stage disease becomes bilateral and bradykinesia increases; consequently, gait is characterized by shuffling steps with increased double limb support, the amplitude of arm swing is additionally reduced and also axial rotation worsens; compare defragmentation of turns, impaired motor automaticity and problems in gait initiation, freezing of gait with risk of falling. In late stage blocks in motor function, fluctuations, and dyskinesias are present and negatively conditioned gait; also muscle endurance and force decline influence gait performances.

Postural instability, due to impairment of postural reflexes, appears in the advanced stages of the disease, with consequent ease of falling, especially following directional changes. To maintain balance, the postural control mechanisms and the maintenance of the center of mass within the support base must be intact. Progressively in patients with Parkinson's disease, these control systems are altered, this leads to an abnormal flexion of the trunk that appears when standing or walking and disappears in the supine position, this is called camptocormia. It is measured by retropulsion or propulsion test (Pull test). This symptom is the most common cause of falls and contributes significantly to the risk of fractures [23]. Apart from the motor symptoms, non-motor symptoms also appear in PD which may result due to the loss of neurons from dopaminergic, non-dopaminergic or a combination of both pathways [24].

The most common neuropsychiatric symptoms that occur in PD are depression, anxiety, phobia, inhibition of social interaction, cognitive impairment, and dementia. Autonomic dysfunctions include blood pressure abnormalities, gastrointestinal dysfunction, sexual abnormalities, thermoregulatory dysfunction, and urinary dysfunction.

The parkinsonian patient has major sleep disorders caused by an alteration of the REM phase. They include the inability to fall asleep or to sleep with frequent nocturnal awakenings (the patient is exhausted in the morning). This creates a lot of discomfort, especially in the family environment. This leads to a possible aggression of care giver. Among sleep disorders, Restless Legs Syndrome (RLS) is a disorder in which the patient feels discomfort in the legs that only subsides when he moves them. Since the disorder improves with dopaminergic therapy, it is believed that it may have a mechanism in common with Parkinson's disease [25].

5. Diagnosis

The diagnosis of Parkinson's disease is predominantly clinical and is based on the presence of the typical characteristics: resting tremor, extrapyramidal rigidity, and bradykinesia. Diagnosis is supported by a good response to dopaminergic therapy and asymmetric limb involvement at onset. The most common diagnostic criteria are those of the United Kingdom Parkinson's Disease Society Brain Bank which identifies:

1. The essential symptoms for the diagnosis of parkinsonian syndrome;
    - Bradykinesia
    - At least one of the following
        - Muscular rigidity
        - 4–6 Hz rest tremor
        - Postural instability not caused by primary visual, vestibular, cerebellar, or proprioceptive dysfunction
2. Exclusion criteria for the diagnosis of Parkinson's disease;
    - History of repeated strokes with stepwise progression of parkinsonian features
    - History of repeated head injury
    - History of definite encephalitis
    - Oculogyric crises

- Neuroleptic treatment at onset of symptoms
- More than one affected relative
- Sustained remission
- Strictly unilateral features after 3 years
- Supranuclear gaze palsy
- Cerebellar signs
- Early severe autonomic involvement
- Early severe dementia with disturbances of memory, language, and praxis
- Babinski sign presence of cerebral tumor or communication hydrocephalus on imaging study
- Negative response to large doses of levodopa in absence of malabsorption
- MPTP exposure

3. Criteria

- Three or more required for diagnosis of definite Parkinson's disease in combination with step one
- Unilateral onset
- Rest tremor present
- Progressive disorder
- Persistent asymmetry affecting side of onset most
- Excellent response (70–100%) to levodopa
- Severe levodopa-induced chorea
- Levodopa response for 5 years or more
- Clinical course of 10 years or more [26].

Instrumental diagnosis is mainly used in cases of atypical Parkinson's and makes use mainly of neuroradiological images: functional magnetic resonance imaging (MRI), also accompanied by nuclear magnetic resonance spectroscopy, and transcranial sonography; a new method that allows the non-invasive and low-cost study of the parenchyma of the basal nuclei and the midbrain, with the help of the temporal window. SPECT and PET tracers can be used with high sensitivity for the assessment of presynaptic dopaminergic deficits. In fact, in 2011, the U.S. Food and Drug Administration approved an imaging scan called the DaTscan or I-123 ioflupane SPECT. This technique allows to see detailed pictures of the brain's dopamine system. Measurement of the dopamine transporter is an indirect indicator of impairment of the dopaminergic system. Tracer uptake in the striatum (yellow and red) is reduced at an early stage of the disease and decreases as the disease progresses [27].

6. Managing symptoms with medication

Pharmacological therapy is based on the use of different strategies, in relation to the various stages of progression of the disease, with the main objective, especially at the beginning, of the Symptom control. In fact, medication administration should begin when patients feel a functional disability. Currently, initial therapy includes the use of carbidopa/levodopa, dopaminergic agonists, monoamine oxidase B (MAO B) inhibitors, anticholinergic agents and amantadine. Treatment is highly individualized and adjusted over time based on symptoms and side effects [28].

7. Rehabilitation

In the literature, there is increasingly solid scientific evidence that confirms the hypothesis of the efficacy of rehabilitation intervention in improving the functional abilities of patients in ADL and the ability to walk (amplitude and speed of the stride) and the overall mobility of patients. Thus was born the concept of—*multidimensional neurorehabilitation* which must be intense as a global and integrated clinical-rehabilitation approach that makes use of all the acquisitions (pharmacological, psychological, rehabilitative) implemented by a multi-specialist team of operators who are also attentive to ethical and relational aspects and who work on shared objectives, aimed at the best use of the patient's residual psychophysical abilities and the achievement of coexistence dignified with illness in an atmosphere of satisfactory quality of life. Rehabilitation interventions represent an alternative strategy to slow or reverse some functional aspects of disability in PD.

A complex sensorimotor rehabilitation protocol could stimulate the glutamate metabolism in basal ganglia and, in turn, neuroplasticity processes. These mechanisms could prepare the ground to restore the functional interaction among brain areas deputed to motor controls, which are affected in PD [29].

The interest in rehabilitation therapy stems from the observation that, despite advances in pharmacological management and new surgical techniques, in a greater number of patients the effect of drugs is gradually reduced with a severe disability, major limitations in the performance of self-care and mobility, and limitation of participation in social activities. Exercise and rehabilitation increase the levels of brain-derived neurotrophic factor and so they determine brain plasticity [30, 31].

Animal studies demonstrate that the neuroprotective and neuro-restorative capacity of intensive exercise and the potential role of exercise in overall brain health may influence the structural (connectivity) and physiological properties of brain function. Many studies have shown that rehabilitation is, particularly, useful as it allows the division of complex motor gestures into segmental movements (in order to gradually recover the totality of automatic motility) so it allows the elaboration of a voluntary motor response aimed at recalling a movement that is difficult to program automatically. One of the techniques used and validated in the scientific field is based on the use of biofeedback. These approaches include conventional rehabilitation training, auditory and visual cueing training and virtual reality training, transcranial direct current stimulation treadmill training.

Progressively, as knowledge of the pathophysiological mechanisms increases, the type of therapeutic approach and exercise to be used to improve the gait of parkinsonian patients has also been defined. The treadmill is a machine for walking or running without moving. This type of training has been used to understand the spinal mechanisms of gait control. Studies carried out on spinalized cats could activate the gait pattern when the hind part of the hind limbs was supported [32, 33]. Therefore, treadmill use was associated with gradual reduction of body weight (BWSTT). The efficacy of BWSTT on gait, balance, and motor function has been demonstrated in several neurological diseases, particularly, stroke and spinal cord injury. In stroke, the authors reported that BWSTT appears as a safe training method, providing an important sense of security regarding falls and facilitating free leg movements, compared to the treadmill alone. It has also been hypothesized that treadmill training promotes a "cortical reorganization," particularly in the supplementary motor area, and that this reorganization may be the basis of the improvements presented by patients. Unlike walking on the floor, where there are oscillations and variability in the characteristics of the step, on the treadmill the patient must follow the speed of movement of the platform, generating a more rhythmic and uniform step. We could, therefore, define the treadmill as an "external gait pacemaker." The progressively more intensive exercise determines a sort of "adaptation" of the patient that improves the control of the automated movement with an increase in proprioceptive perception of the step and voluntary awareness of the exercise. A Cochrane review found that the use of treadmill training in patients with Parkinson's disease can significantly improve both walking speed and stride width. Numerous studies show that BWSTT improves the general motor performance of patients with Parkinson's disease, in particular: it improves muscle strength, balance, postural instability, and walking speed and reduces the risk of falls, improves quality of life [34].

In PD, many data in the literature show how treadmill training, acting as a sensory cue, improves kinetic and kinematic parameters, studied with computerized gait analysis (CGA), more than physiotherapy alone. There are different methods to achieve a specific motor task in the reinforced environment such as virtual reality, gaming exercise, dual-task and auditory and visual cueing [35, 36].

Many studies demonstrated that rhythmic auditory stimulation (RAS) can improve gait in PD patients. For example, walking with a metronome can improve walking speed and stride length and reduce timing variability [37].

In recent years, neurorehabilitation research has been concerned about virtual reality (VR) as a therapeutic tool. In terms of kinematics learning, VR allows for high-intensity, task-oriented and multi-sensory feedback training that can enhance patients' visual, auditory, and tactile input by making them experience either immersive or non-immersive virtual environments to increase their interests in the entire rehabilitation process, thus enhancing their adherence to treatment [38]. Stroke, cognitive function, and quality of life in the elderly have all been extensively studied with regards to VR technology. Besides, it is also found that postural control function and activity of daily living (ADL) are enhanced following VR intervention [39]. However, the Cochrane Library systematic review showed that only stride speed and stride length were positively affected by VR rehabilitation exercise compared with traditional physical therapy in PD patients. The inconsistent results are due to few studies conducted on a small sample size subjected to VR rehabilitation training. It is still not clear whether this new development will be beneficial or harmful for individuals suffering from Parkinson's disease [13, 40].

Exergames are computer games that are driven by the gross physical movements of the player. They work by combining real-time motion detection with an exciting video game that motivates people to exercise. Exergaming as a therapeutic tool involves functional, targeted, and exciting exercises in a quantifiable and reliable manner. Recent evidence in older adults suggests that playing exergames may also improve cognitive function [41]. Thus, exergaming could be a cost-effective, home-based tool to complement traditional motor symptom rehabilitation in patients with PD. The role of exergaming in PD is represented especially in improving balance and gait [42].

Furthermore, among the technologies used in rehabilitation there is growing interest in using robot-assisted gait training (RAGT) as a novel PT technique in PD [43]. Robotic gait training (RAGT) devices, by definition, transmit the energy required to enable lower limb movement and typically use actuators or motors [44]. These devices are designed to physically guide repetitive, rhythmic bilateral movements of the lower limbs to produce a more normal gait cycle. The provision of a constant stride length and continuous, multimodal rhythmic external stimulation appears to be a valid alternative. RAGT has shown several benefits for gait in PD and may help improve walking ability in dual-task cognitive impairment. However, the important changes in therapeutic mechanisms and functional connectivity associated with RAGT and associated with improved functional gait may complement traditional treatment strategies [45].

8. Instrumental physical therapy

Focused mechano-acoustic vibration was administered by means of Vibration Sound System®. It consists of a 32,000-revolution turbine with a flow rate of 35 m^3/hour able to generate airwaves with a pressure up to 250 mbar, and of a flow modulator that makes the air vibrate with a pressure up to 630 mbar and a frequency up to 980 Hz (however, frequency within 300 Hz) [46].

This new form of energy enables us to re-establish and maintain coordination between sensory information and neuromuscular system hence successfully restoring muscular strength and tone. Unlike the traditional WBV plates, this modified acoustic wave assumes an enlarged sinusoidal periodic waveform similar to a square-wave type where its amplitude changes over at a specific frequency between fixed minimum and maximum values with equal durations for both the minimums as well as maximums while the transition from one extreme to another is instantaneous. In this way, it is possible to instantly reach the maximum amplitude of oscillations and keep it constant or regularly stimulate Pacinian corpuscles (the most important vibratory receptors) within the entire period of its stimulus [47–49]. In Parkinson's disease, the use of Sinergy Viss determines a modulation of muscle tone, allows an improvement of dystonia and rigidity of antigravity muscles and together with treadmill training induces brain plasticity of brain areas deputed to motor controls, which are affected in PD [29].

9. Observation therapy

Action Observation Therapy (AOT) is a multidisciplinary approach from neuroscience that involves somatosensory and cognitive recovery. This pathway works by activating the brain's mirror neuron (MNS) [50, 51]. This helps plan movement and neuroplasticity. A combination of practices (apps) have promising strategies to promote physical activity and maintain functional capacity in PD. Therefore, this therapy can improve the motor functions of the limbs and activities of daily living such as eating, washing, and using dishes [52].

10. Microgravity aquatic therapy

Microgravity aquatic therapy is based on several important biotechnological properties. The fundamental forces acting on a patient immersed in water consist of buoyancy forces, resistance, and inertia. Other factors that affect the patient include hydrostatic pressure and heat. Rehabilitation pools have a temperature of about 30–33°C. Several properties of water contribute to its therapeutic effects, such as the ability to use water for strength instead of gravity or weight, thermal stability, temperature is almost constant. Hydrostatic pressure also supports, stabilizes, and influences heart and lung function. The hydrostatic force allows you to float and reduces the effects of gravity. Turbulence and wave propagation of the fluid allow for smooth maneuvering and movement. Through therapy in an aquatic microgravity environment, it is possible to adjust the intensity of the exercise, the resistance of the water changes depending on the walking speed. In fact, slow movements such as walking, movements that require a large amount of muscle strength in a short period of time, experience increased water resistance [53]. Previous studies have shown that exercising in water, where buoyancy makes it difficult to support the body, reduces postural instability and improves dynamic balance and muscle strength. In fact, water aerobics is widely used in the rehabilitation of neurological diseases [54–56] and refers to water aerobics or rehabilitation training and treatment methods that can reduce patients' symptoms and improve their fitness functions. It can effectively improve balance, walking ability, and quality of life in patients with Parkinson's disease.

11. Speech therapy and treatment of dysphagia

Speech therapists can help people with Parkinson's disease to communicate as much as possible. They also teach nonverbal communication as well as energy conservation. Dysphagia, or difficulty swallowing, will often occur at some point in the disease process. It is important to recognize these signs to ensure safety with meals and medications. Some signs of dysphagia may include an increase in coughing or choking during meals, throat clearing or feeling foods "get stuck" in the throat after swallowing. It is important to further assess swallowing function with the assistance of an SLP to determine the safest and least restrictive diet recommendations and provide appropriate exercises to improve swallow function. The VitalStim® System can be used for PD. It is a painless non-invasive therapy for treating dysphagia, obtained by external electrical stimulation which is applied to the front of the neck (defined as such in the market by the Food and Drug Administration in 2002). It provides neuromuscular electrical stimulation (NMES) of the involved muscles to improve the function of swallowing [57].

12. Psychological therapy

Parkinson's disease is related to changes in neurotransmitters in the brain, which can result in depression, anxiety, and even hallucinations. Furthermore, cognitive changes associated with Parkinson's disease can range from mild problems (that do not impair day-to-day tasks) to dementia. There are three cognitive areas that are most frequently impacted by Parkinson's disease: executive functioning, attention, memory. Psychologists play a critical role in the interdisciplinary care team for Parkinson's disease, addressing the psychological, emotional, and cognitive needs of individuals with the condition and their caregivers, and promoting overall well-being and quality of life. Neuropsychologists can evaluate changes in mood and/or cognition (including executive functioning, processing speed, and attention) and make treatment recommendations in order to maximize the patient's strengths [58].

13. Complementary therapy

Various complementary therapies are suggested for individuals with PD, typically categorized as dietary, nutritional, and physical [59].

In fact, in recent years, therapeutic proposals have expanded their frontiers, such as music therapy, dance therapy, theater and tai chi (taiji), Nordic walking. Some people with Parkinson's and their family and carers have found complementary therapies useful. It also improves posture, coordination, rhythm, and breathing and prevents falls [60].

14. Conclusions

Rehabilitation plays an important role in the treatment of Parkinson's disease (PD). Numerous studies have addressed the issue of the effectiveness of rehabilitation intervention in Parkinson's disease with a marked increase in the number of publications since the 2000s. The expression of this pathology resulting from the interaction of motor and non-motor symptoms can be extremely variable and make patient management very complex so a multidisciplinary and rehabilitative management of patients with Parkinson's Disease is important. The rehabilitation approach must be a multidisciplinary Parkinson's Disease Multimodal Complex Treatment.

Conflict of interest

The authors declare no conflict of interest.

Author details

Simona Maria Carmignano[1,2]

1 Department of Medicine, Surgery and Dentistry "Salernitan Medical School", University of Salerno, Baronissi, Italy

2 C.T.R. Rehabilitation Therapeutic Center, Tramutola, Basilicata, Italy

*Address all correspondence to: simona.carmignano@gmail.com

References

[1] Von Campenhausen S, Bornschein B, Wick R, Bötzel K, Sampaio C, Poewe W, et al. Prevalence and incidence of Parkinson's disease in Europe. European Neuropsychopharmacology. 2005;**15**:473-490

[2] Parkinson J. An essay on the shaking palsy. The Journal of Neuropsychiatry and Clinical Neurosciences. 2002;**14**(2):223-236

[3] Frenkel-Toledo S, Giladi N, Peretz C, Herman T, Gruendlinger L, Hausdorff JM. Treadmill walking as an external pacemaker to improve gait rhythm and stability in Parkinson's disease. Movement Disorders. 2005;**20**(9):1109-1114. DOI: 10.1002/mds.20507

[4] Mak MK, Pang MY, Mok V. Gait difficulty, postural instability, and muscle weakness are associated with fear of falling in people with Parkinson's disease. Parkinson's Disease. 2012;**2012**:901721. DOI: 10.1155/2012/901721. Epub 2011 Oct 5

[5] Mirelman A, Bonato P, Camicioli R, Ellis TD, Giladi N, Hamilton JL, et al. Gait impairments in Parkinson's disease. Lancet Neurology. 2019;**18**:697-708

[6] Frazzitta G. Rehabilitation and Parkinson's disease: A happy marriage! International Journal of Physical Medicine and Rehabilitation. 2013;**1**:2. DOI: 10.4172/2329-9096.1000109

[7] Katzenschlager R, Lees AJ. Treatment of Parkinson's disease: Levodopa as the first choice. Journal of Neurology. 2002;**249**:II19-II24

[8] Rajput AH, Offord KP, Beard CM, Kurland LT. Epidemiology of parkinsonism: Incidence, classification, and mortality. Annals of Neurology. 1984;**16**(3):278-282

[9] Ben-Shlomo Y, Darweesh S, Llibre-Guerra J, et al. The epidemiology of Parkinson's disease. Lancet. 2024;**403**:283-292

[10] Penney JB Jr, Young AB. Striatal inhomogeneities and basal ganglia function. Movement Disorders. 1986;**1**:3-15

[11] Bastian AJ, Kelly VE, Perlmutter JS, Mink JW. Effects of pallidotomy and levodopa on walking and reaching movements in Parkinson's disease. Movement Disorders: Official Journal of the Movement Disorder Society. 2003;**18**(9):1008-1017

[12] Schultz W. Multiple dopamine functions at different time courses. Annual Review of Neuroscience. 2007;**30**:259-288. DOI: 10.1146/annurev.neuro.28.061604.135722

[13] Bauer ACM, Andringa G. The potential of immersive virtual reality for cognitive training in elderly. Gerontology. 2020;**66**(6):614-623

[14] Sandyk R, Iacono RP, Bamford CR. The hypothalamus in Parkinson disease. Italian Journal of Neurological Sciences. 1987;**8**:227-234. DOI: 10.1007/BF02337479

[15] Hoehn MM, Yahr MD. Parkinsonism: Onset, progression, and mortality. Neurology. 2001;**57**(10 Suppl. 3):S11-S26

[16] Bateson MC, Gibberd FB, Wilson RSE. Salivary symptoms in Parkinson's disease. Archives of Neurology. 1973;**29**:274-275

[17] Altmann LJP, Troche MS. High-level language production in Parkinson's disease: A review. Parkinson's Disease. 2011;**2011**:1-12. DOI: 10.4061/2011/238956

[18] Gunnery SD, Habermann B, Saint-Hilaire M, Thomas CA, Tickle-Degnen L. The relationship between the experience of hypomimia and social wellbeing in people with Parkinson's disease and their care partners. Journal of Parkinson's Disease. 2016;**6**(3):625-630. DOI: 10.3233/JPD-160782

[19] Jankovic J, Williams L, Wilkins Tolosa E, Jankovic J, Fahn S. Parkinson's Disease and Movement Disorders. 4th ed. Philadelphia: Dystonic; 2002

[20] Plotnik M, Giladi N, Hausdorff JM. Is freezing of gait in Parkinson's disease a result of multiple gait impairments? Implications for treatment. Parkinson's Disease. 2012;**2012**:459321

[21] Bartels AL, Balash Y, Gurevich T, Schaafsma JD, Hausdorff JM, Giladi NJ. Relationship between freezing of gait (FOG) and other features of Parkinson's: FOG is not correlated with bradykinesia. Clinical Neuroscience. 2003;**10**(5):584-588

[22] Giladi N, Shabtai H, Rozenberg E, Shabtai E. Gait festination in Parkinson's disease. Parkinsonism & Related Disorders. 2001;7:135-138

[23] Bloch F, Houeto JL, Tezenas du Montcel S, Bonneville F, Etchepare F, Welter ML, et al. Parkinson's disease with camptocormia. Journal of Neurology, Neurosurgery, and Psychiatry. 2006;77(11):1223-1228. DOI: 10.1136/jnnp.2006.087908. Epub 2006 Jun 5

[24] Todorova A, Jenner P, Ray Chaudhuri K. Non-motor Parkinson's: Integral to motor Parkinson's, yet often neglected. Practical Neurology. 2014;**14**(5):310-322. DOI: 10.1136/practneurol-2013-000741. Epub 2014 Apr 3

[25] Martinez-Martin P, Chaudhuri KR, Rojo-Abuin JM, Rodriguez-Blazquez C, Alvarez-Sanchez M, Arakaki T, et al. Assessing the non-motor symptoms of Parkinson's disease: MDS-UPDRS and NMS scale. European Journal of Neurology. 2015;**22**(1):37-43. DOI: 10.1111/ene.12165. Epub 2013 Apr 22

[26] Gibb WR, Lees AJ. The relevance of the Lewy body to the pathogenesis of idiopathic Parkinson's disease. Journal of Neurology, Neurosurgery, and Psychiatry. 1988;**51**(06):745-752

[27] Patel KP, Wymer DT, Bhatia VK, Duara R, Rajadhyaksha CD. Multimodality imaging of dementia: Clinical importance and role of integrated anatomic and molecular imaging. RadioGraphics. 2020;**40**(1):200-222. DOI: 10.1148/rg.2020190070

[28] Connolly BS, Lang AE. Pharmacological treatment of Parkinson disease: A review. JAMA. 2014;**311**(16):1670-1683

[29] Delli Pizzi S, Bellomo RG, Carmignano SM, Ancona E, Franciotti R, Supplizi M, et al. Rehabilitation program based on sensorimotor recovery improves the static and dynamic balance and modifies the basal ganglia neurochemistry: A pilot 1H-MRS study on Parkinson's disease patients. Medicine (Baltimore). 2017;**96**(50):e8732. DOI: 10.1097/MD.0000000000008732

[30] Ahlskog JE. Does vigorous exercise have a neuroprotective effect in Parkinson disease? Neurology. 2011;**77**(3):288-294

[31] Hirsch MA, Iyer SS, Sanjak M. Exercise-induced neuroplasticity in human Parkinson's disease: What is the evidence telling us? Parkinsonism & Related Disorders. 2016;**22** (Suppl. 1):S78-S81

[32] Lovely RG, Gregor RJ, Roy RR, Edgerton VR. Effects of training on the recovery of full weight-bearing stepping in the adult spinal cat. Experimental Neurology. 1986;**92**:421-435

[33] Earhart GM, Williams AJ. Treadmill training for individuals with Parkinson disease. Physical Therapy. 2012;**92**(7):893-897. DOI: 10.2522/ptj.20110471

[34] Mehrholz J, Kugler J, Storch A, Pohl M, Hirsch K, Elsner B. Treadmill training for patients with Parkinson's disease. Cochrane Database of Systematic Reviews. 2015;**13**(9):CD007830. DOI: 10.1002/14651858.CD007830

[35] Morris ME. Movement disorders in people with Parkinson disease: A model for physical therapy. Physical Therapy. 2000;**80**(6):578-597

[36] Petzinger GM, Fisher BE, McEwen S, Beeler JA, Walsh JP, Jakowec MW. Exercise-enhanced neuroplasticity targeting motor and cognitive circuitry in Parkinson's disease. Lancet Neurology. 2013;**12**(7):716-726. DOI: 10.1016/S1474-4422(13)70123-6

[37] Ashoori A, Eagleman DM, Jankovic J. Effects of auditory rhythm and music on gait disturbances in Parkinson's disease. Frontiers in Neurology. 2015;**6**:234. DOI: 10.3389/fneur.2015.00234

[38] Canning CG et al. Virtual reality in research and rehabilitation of gait and balance in Parkinson disease. Nature Reviews Neurology. 2020;**16**(8):409-425

[39] Laver KE, Lange B, George S, Deutsch JE, Saposnik G, Crotty M. Virtual reality for stroke rehabilitation. Cochrane Database of Systematic Reviews. 20 Nov 2017;**11**(11):CD008349. DOI: 10.1002/14651858.CD008349.pub4

[40] Lei C, Sunzi K, Dai F, Liu X, Wang Y, Zhang B, et al. Effects of virtual reality rehabilitation training on gait and balance in patients with Parkinson's disease: A systematic review. PLoS ONE. 2019;**14**(11):e0224819

[41] Padala KP, Padala PR, Burke WJ. Wii-fit as an adjunct for mild cognitive impairment: Clinical perspectives. Journal of the American Geriatrics Society. 2011;**59**:932-933

[42] Barry G, Galna B, Rochester L. The role of exergaming in Parkinson's disease rehabilitation: A systematic review of the evidence. Journal of Neuroengineering and Rehabilitation. 2014;**11**:1-10

[43] Alwardat M, Etoom M, Al Dajah S, Schirinzi T, Di Lazzaro G, Salimei PS, et al. Effectiveness of robot-assisted gait training on motor impairments in people with Parkinson's disease: A systematic review and meta-analysis. International Journal of Rehabilitation Research. 2018;**41**(4):287-296

[44] Banala SK et al. Robot assisted gait training with active leg exoskeleton (ALEX). IEEE Transactions on Neural Systems and Rehabilitation Engineering. 2008;**17**(1):2-8

[45] Carmignano SM et al. Robot-assisted gait training in patients with Parkinson's disease: Implications for clinical practice. A systematic review. Neuropsychological Rehabilitation. 2022;**51**(4):649-663

[46] Saggini R, Ancona E, Carmignano SM, Supplizi M, Barassi G, Bellomo RG. Effect of combined treatment

with focused mechano-acoustic vibration and pharmacological therapy on bone mineral density and muscle strength in post-menopausal women. Clinical Cases in Mineral and Bone Metabolism. 2017;**14**(3):305-311. DOI: 10.11138/ccmbm/2017.14.3.305. Epub 2017 Dec 27

[47] Saggini R, Di Stefano A, Capogrosso F, Carmignano SM, D'Ettole S, Iodice P, et al. Task-oriented physical exercise using postural re-alignment with body weight support in chronic stroke. European Journal of Inflammation. 2013;**11**(3):739-749

[48] Constantino C, Galuppo L, Romiti D. Efficacy of mechano-acoustic vibration on strength, pain, and function in poststroke rehabilitation: A pilot study. Topics in Stroke Rehabilitation. 2014;**21**(5):391-399

[49] Bellomo RG, Di Pancrazio L, Khodor H, Saggini R, Barassi G, Carmignano SM, et al. Global bioprogressive rehabilitation program and postural instability in Parkinson's disease. European Scientific Journal. June 2014/SPECIAL/edition Vol. 2. pp. 310-321. ISSN: 1857-7881 (Print) e-ISSN 1857-7431

[50] Johansson BB. Current trends in stroke rehabilitation. A review with focus on brain plasticity. Acta Neurologica Scandinavica. 2011;**123**(3):147-159

[51] Shih TY, Wu CY, Lin KC, Cheng CH, Hsieh YW, Chen CL, et al. Effects of action observation therapy and mirror therapy after stroke on rehabilitation outcomes and neural mechanisms by MEG: Study protocol for a randomized controlled trial. Trials. 2017;**18**(1):459

[52] Ge S, Liu H, Lin P, Gao J, Xiao C, Li Z. Neural basis of action observation and understanding from first-and third-person perspectives: An fMRI study. Frontiers in Behavioral Neuroscience. 2018;**12**:283

[53] Barassi G, Bellomo RG, Porreca A, Giannuzzo G, Irace G, Trivisano L, et al. Rehabilitation of Neuromotor Disabilities in Aquatic Microgravity Environment. In: Respiratory Ailments in Context. Advances in Experimental Medicine, Biology - Neuroscience and Respiration. Springer International Publishing AG; 2018. pp. 61-73. DOI: 10.1007/5584_2018_164

[54] Castro-Sánchez AM et al. Hydrotherapy for the treatment of pain in people with multiple sclerosis: A randomized controlled trial. Evidence-Based Complementary and Alternative Medicine. 2012;**2012**(1):473963

[55] Marinho-Buzelli AR et al. The use of aquatic therapy among rehabilitation professionals for individuals with spinal cord injury or disorder. The Journal of Spinal Cord Medicine. 2019;**42** (Suppl. 1):158-165

[56] Saleh MSM, Rehab NI, Aly SMA. Effect of aquatic versus land motor dual task training on balance and gait of patients with chronic stroke: A randomized controlled trial. NeuroRehabilitation. 2019;**44**(4):485-492

[57] Farooq N, Khatoon S, Malik AN, Rathore FA. Role of Vitalstim® in the management of patients with dysphagia: A minireview. The Journal of the Pakistan Medical Association. 2023;**73**(6):1346-1348. DOI: 10.47391/JPMA.23-46

[58] Zarotti N, Eccles FJR, Foley JA, Paget A, Gunn S, Leroi I, et al. Psychological interventions for people with Parkinson's disease in the early 2020s: Where do we stand? Psychology

and Psychotherapy. 2021;**94**(3):760-797. DOI: 10.1111/papt.12321. Epub 2020 Nov 11

[59] Zesiewicz TA, Evatt ML. Potential influences of complementary therapy on motor and non-motor complications in Parkinson's disease. CNS Drugs. 2009;**23**:817-835

[60] Deuel LM, Seeberger LC. Complementary therapies in Parkinson disease: A review of acupuncture, Tai Chi, Qi Gong, Yoga, and Cannabis. Neurotherapeutics. 2020;**17**:1434-1455. DOI: 10.1007/s13311-020-00900-y

Chapter 9

The Effects of Neurofeedback Training in Patients with Parkinson's Disease

Valeska Kouzak, Maria Clotilde Tavares and Wendy Isabel Silvestre da Silva

Abstract

Parkinson's disease (PD) is the second most prevalent degenerative disorder impacting the central nervous system. PD manifests through both motor and non-motor symptoms, including rest tremors, bradykinesia, muscle rigidity, neuropsychiatric distress, anosmia, and deficits in executive function and memory. Neurofeedback (NFB) is a psychophysiological technique aimed at enabling individuals to self-regulate their brain activity by utilizing instruments that provide real-time feedback on cerebral activity. The present chapter aims to state the theory that has been produced about Neurofeedback in Parkinson's disease. To achieve that, firstly, the conceptualization of PD has been made; secondly, the neuropsychological and neuropsychiatric symptoms were described; thirdly, the neurophysiology of PD was presented; and finally, the neurofeedback applied in PD was analyzed. Most of the studies are related to the improvement of motor performance, although the non-motor symptoms might be another aim to improve the quality of life of those patients.

Keywords: EEG, neuropsychiatry, neuropsychology, neuromodulation, SMR

1. Introduction

Parkinson's disease (PD) is a central nervous system progressive pathology and the second most common degenerative disease in the world. It occurs in one to two individuals for each 1000 in the general population [1]. The PD prevalence reflects the incidence and the duration of pathology. The incidence of PD is connected to protective and risk factors, in which the higher risk factor is age, followed by chemical products and pollutants such as pesticides, solvents and heavy metals. On the other side, smoking is associated with lower risks of PD, but this causal association is debatable [2].

The most common PD symptoms that characterize it differently from other progressive pathologies are bradykinesia, muscle rigidity, resting tremor, and postural instability [3]. However, not only motor symptoms affect the quality-of-life of

 IntechOpen

individuals with PD but also non-motor symptoms such as anosmia, constipation, and neuropsychiatric alterations are part of the disease characteristics [4], as well as cognitive loss [5].

The physiopathology of PD implies the degeneration of dopaminergic nigrostriatal circuits, characterized by motor alterations, and the α-synuclein protein neuronal deposit under the form of Lewy body, involving other cerebral areas beyond the *substantia nigra* of the mesencephalic region, with the commitment of non-dopaminergic neurons [6].

According to the Braak theory [7] PD presents six degenerative stages linked to α-synuclein deletion in the brain; briefly, it can describe an evolution of pathology in the following way: firstly α-synuclein aggregate in the nervous system appears in the interior of olfactive structures and the motor dorsal nucleus of the vagus nerve, followed by the inferior portion of the Rafe Nuclei and the Locus Coeruleus in the second stage. Only at the third stage that the *substantia nigra* is affected together with the amygdala, integumentary pedunculopontine nucleus, and the superior portion of Rafe Nuclei, among other areas. During the fourth stage α-synuclein spreads to hippocampal formation and cortical-specific areas, and finally, in the last two stages [5, 6], almost the entire cortex is injured [8].

Moreover, patients with PD also present degeneration in many other neuronal systems including the locus coeruleus noradrenergic pathway, the motor vagal nuclei, the serotoninergic pathway of the Rafe nucleus, the cholinergic pathway of the nucleus basalis of Meynert, pedunculopontine nucleus, Edinger-Westphal nucleus, and other brainstem nuclei [9], in which some of these pathways have influenced the symptoms composition.

Therefore, it is well known that the propagation of α-synuclein in the brain occurs in stages and that the injury to other areas precedes the neuron degeneration of *substantia nigra*, affecting glutamatergic, noradrenergic, serotoninergic, histaminergic, and cholinergic projections [10].

According to the canonic model [11], the dopaminergic circuit alterations in direction to the striated body in receptors D1 (excitatory) and D2 (inhibitory) provoke an irregular neuronal communication in the thalamic pathway. Therefore, according to this model, the imbalance in the activity of these two neuronal pathways, that is, direct and indirect, resulting from the dopaminergic denervation is responsible for generating the bradykinesia and stiffness. Thus, the *substantia nigra pars compacta* neurons (SNpc) arouse the excitatory pathway D1, that is, arouse the direct pathway and inhibit the receptors D2 from the indirect pathway, respectively, in segregated classes of medial spine neurons (MSN), which forms the only way out of the striate body. Besides that, the MSN sends projections to pale globe *pars interna* (GPi) and the pale globe *pars externa* (GPe). The GPi functions as the primary output nucleus of the basal ganglia, sending continuous inhibitory signals to the thalamus. As a result, the thalamus transmits excitatory signals to the neocortex, completing the thalamocortical loop of the basal nuclei. This loop forms a dense glutamatergic pathway of afferent innervation from the striatum, contributing to the neurophysiological changes that will be discussed further.

Due to PD being a degenerative pathology of the central nervous system, there is no definitive cure for their symptoms. However, the disease presents a positive response to medication—levodopa—a substance that acts in the dopaminergic pathway, replacing the dopamine production in the affected neurons, although its action does not prevent the continuous degeneration of brain areas and other resources are needed to control the pathology [3].

An alternative to regulate movement in advanced stages or with lower response to medication is Deep Brain Stimulation—DBS, as it produces electricity in the affected region, providing an inhibitory action of the region, similar to a thalamotomy or ablation, however reversible and controllable [12].

The DBS involves risks, that is, a surgical and invasive procedure with side effects; besides, with time, its action might decline because of the degeneration [13]. Moreover, another alternative to resistant medication cases, that has been used to treat motor symptoms in PD, is the Guided Focus Ultrasound-MRI which consists of beam emission by magnetic resonance in order to promote the ablation of the thalamic region precisely increasing the region temperature leading to a neuronal lesion. The ultrasound technique has been applied since the 80s but has only become frequent in the last few years, mainly because of the magnetic resonance technology, which supports the provision of a non-invasive procedure without cutting [14].

Therefore, alternatives that favor the improvement of motor function and the diminishing of affective and cognitive disability are important ways to improve the quality of life in PD patients.

2. Neuropsychological changes in Parkinson's disease

The PD presents several motor and non-motor symptoms, including neuropsychological aspects, which will be detailed in this section. According to Luria [15], neuropsychology has the purpose of investigating the role of specific brain systems in the complex form of mental activity, that is, the union between cognitive process—perception, attention, memory, reasoning, emotion, language, planning, and motor control—and neuroscience—how the nervous system act in its function and organization [16, 17].

Consequently, as PD presents neuronal degeneration in several pathways and progressively modifies individual mental activity, it has a series of neuropsychological symptoms that must be addressed, starting from the motor symptom itself. The degeneration of basal ganglia occurs because the dopaminergic neuronal loss at the *substantia nigra pars compacta* affects the inhibitory pathway leading to the pathology's most characteristic symptom, which is freezing or tremor, that is, the neuronal consequence over movement. Moreover, physiologically, the cortex keeps the action planning at the premotor and motor region in the frontal lobe; however, the abnormal neuronal function of the basal ganglia affects the velocity to initiate the movement, which remains slowed during action performance [16]. Consequently, these two examples represent the first recognized neuropsychological impairment of PD, that is, motor control.

Besides that, the PD diagnostic evolution from observation of other symptoms and with the detailed physiopathology, including non-motor symptoms, brought light to new perspectives on the pathology [18].

Therefore, other neurocognitive disorders are observed as common features of PD, with the consequence of a prevalence of dementia in 26% of the cases in the initial phase and longitudinally that of 78.2% of dementia cases in 8 years after diagnosis [19]. Moreover, the prevalence of cognitive decline in non-dementia patients is 25% [20]. The common pattern of cognitive alterations in PD is the dysexecutive syndrome, despite the fact that a variety of visuospatial, memory, and language deficits has been observed [21].

Based on the diversity of PD manifestations, there have been proposed that cognitive difficulties are the result of two syndromes that partially overcome. One is related to dopaminergic loss of the basal pathways leading to attentional and executive deficits, and the other is in the posterior region associated with the cholinergic degeneration with cognitive loss associated with the cortical posterior bases, that is, recognition memory and visuospatial skills deficits. Therefore, it has been called "Dual syndrome," in which the cognitive deficits are specific domain, frontal striatal and/or cortical posterior [22].

A study conducted by Barvas et al. [23] evaluated 65 patients in their neuropsychological function in order to check the cognitive phenotype pattern of PD, in which they present a qualitative description of three groups. Group A, 21.54%, includes patients with no cognitive deficits or a mild difficulty in memory and executive function and those with performance in attention, visual and verbal long-term memory, executive function, social cognition, language, and visuospatial skills better than the other two groups. Group B includes 53.85% of the sample and is composed of patients with intermediate cognitive impairments and significantly lower scores than group A in attention, episodic memory, social cognition, and verbal fluency, not presenting a significant difference in executive function and tests of naming than group A.

At last, group C represents 24.61% of the sample, which includes patients with higher cognitive impairments, with lower performance compared to group A in all tests, and higher deficits compared to group B in executive function and visuospatial skills. According to the "Dual syndrome" hypothesis, it might be said that group A and B reflects the difference in the degree of cognitive symptoms associated with dopaminergic loss over the basal ganglia pathway, and group C reflects the cognitive symptoms associated with the cortical degeneration of cholinergic loss. Alternatively, the difference observed in group B might be associated with symptoms regarding dopaminergic loss and the initial corticoposterior degeneration.

Besides that, the study also observed a difference between groups B and C in relation to education, in which group B had more years of study than group C, that is, an indicative of cognitive reserve in this group, once the number of education year is one of the factors for cognitive reserve, contributing to executive functions and memory in patients with PD [24].

No other demographic difference or clinic was found between groups; therefore, gender, time of disease, severity of motor incapacity, as well as depression and anxiety did not interfere with cognitive capacity; however, there was a relationship between daily living activity and cognitive performance, once there was a difference between groups in this area, in which group C had lower scores compared to group A [23].

In general, we can differentiate brain atrophy in Parkinson's disease when it occurs with dementia (PDD) and with mild cognitive impairment (MCI) associated with PD. Therefore, there are atrophy patterns that can be summarized as follows:

PDD:

- More pronounced bilateral gray matter atrophy in the medial frontal region, right precuneus, left inferior parietal lobe, left superior frontal gyrus, and left middle temporal gyrus [25].
- Atrophy in the occipital lobes is more intense than in PD without dementia [26].
- Atrophy of the hippocampus and entorhinal cortex is less pronounced than in Alzheimer's disease (AD) [27].

MCI:

- Atrophy of the occipito-temporal cortex (fusiform gyrus) in cases with facial recognition deficits.
- Atrophied parietal areas in cases with deficits in visual shape discrimination [28].
- Atrophy of the non-dominant extra-striate visual cortex in cases with stereopsis deficits [29–31].
- Cortical thinning identifiable before the diagnosis of MCI [32].
- More accelerated cortical thinning in the left middle frontal gyrus, right superior frontal gyrus, and left superior temporal gyrus [33, 34].
- Smaller volumes of the left nucleus accumbens, left caudate, and hippocampus [29, 35, 36].

Thus, the correlations between degenerative changes and cognitive performance can be defined as follows:

- Striatum: Lower performance in phonemic verbal fluency.
- Right parietal cortex: Better performance in visual memory-free recall.
- Central portion of the corpus callosum: Performance in attention/working memory.
- Mid-posterior region of the corpus callosum: Executive functions, language, and memory.
- Posterior section of the corpus callosum: Memory and visuospatial domains.

Furthermore, imaging biomarkers are currently being used to examine the expansion of the lateral ventricles and atrophy of the corpus callosum. Therefore, when it comes to PDD and MCI, brain atrophy presents distinct patterns, with different brain regions being affected in each case. Nonetheless, it can still be a useful biomarker for diagnosing and monitoring disease progression [37].

3. Neuropsychiatric disorders associated with Parkinson's disease

Parkinson's disease (PD) also presents neuropsychiatric symptoms among its non-motor symptoms in comorbidity with the progression of the pathology, with the most frequent being anxiety, depression, apathy, and psychosis, occurring in most patients at some point during the course of pathology. The symptoms mentioned above are among the most important to be considered in PD as they directly affect the patient's quality of life [38].

The two most common neuropsychiatric disorders are depression and anxiety, with approximately 30–40% of PD patients having significant symptoms of depression and anxiety affecting about 40% of patients with PD. The symptoms of both neuropsychiatric pathologies can be related to periods off medication, which usually, but not always, seem to follow motor fluctuations and respond well to antiparkinsonian medication [39].

Both depression and anxiety can occur several years before motor symptoms, being considered one of the prodromal non-motor symptoms of the pathology [40].

Anxiety is the most common neuropsychiatric symptom, affecting about 31% of PD patients, according to the study by Kalia and Lang [41]. Another recent study suggests that anxiety in PD may be associated with a reduction in cognitive control of emotional processes [42], becoming a burden for these patients as it may be associated with motor disability and reduced quality of life [43].

Garlovsky et al. [44] identified that personality traits, coping style, social support, and pathology are psychosocial predictors of anxiety in PD. Additionally, individuals with avoidant or pessimistic personality traits are associated with higher levels of anxiety, mainly because they are less competent in dealing with negative emotional experiences. On the other hand, social support and a sense of identity seem to be protective mechanisms.

A systematic review by Carey et al. [45] demonstrated that anxiety associated with Parkinson's disease (PD) is linked to structural and functional changes in the cortico-striato-thalamo-cortical (CSTC) limbic circuit and the fear circuit. Consequently, anxiety in PD may result from an imbalance between these two circuits.

Furthermore, the shared pathophysiology between anxiety and PD may account for the shared symptoms between the two conditions. The dopaminergic theory indicates that mesolimbic and mesocortical neurodegeneration of dopaminergic projections observed as early changes in PD is highly associated with anxiety in PD [46].

The depletion of serotonergic nerve cells in the raphe nuclei [47] results in increased anxiety symptoms in PD patients [48]. And the degeneration of the locus coeruleus, rich in norepinephrine, is responsible for generating physiological anxiety reactions [49]. Consequently, the deficits of these neurotransmitters also lead to a high frequency of anxiety in PD.

Moreover, there is an overlap of anxiety and PD symptoms, meaning behavioral changes associated with anxiety can be similar to PD physical symptoms. For example, agitation can be confused with tremors, restlessness and dyskinesia. Conversely, symptoms associated with PD can resemble anxiety, such as muscle tension, fatigue, and difficulty concentrating. Thus, these symptoms can be confusing in determining whether patients are experiencing anxiety or PD symptoms [50], making differential diagnosis based on observed symptoms difficult.

In the case of depression, differential diagnosis difficulties are also observed since, despite the key characteristics of depression being low mood and lack of interest or pleasure (anhedonia), changes in sleep, appetite, loss of libido, psychomotor retardation, reduced memory, and loss of energy are characteristics that can overlap with PD symptoms [51].

Similar to what occurs with anxiety, many neurobiological findings have shown that depression in PD may not only result from deficiencies in serotonergic pathways but also from reduced dopaminergic and noradrenergic innervation in the limbic and striatal systems [52]. Consistently, depression in PD can be treated using selective serotonin reuptake inhibitors, serotonin/norepinephrine reuptake inhibitors, and dopaminergic agonists [53] in conjunction with antiparkinsonian medications.

Mesolimbic dopaminergic denervation plays a crucial role in the development of apathy and depression, potentially explaining the frequent comorbidity observed in

PD patients. There is confirmed evidence that dopaminergic agonists can improve depression and apathy in Parkinson's patients [54, 55], which is consistent with the fact that depression and apathy are conceptualized as hypodopaminergic syndromes related to PD.

However, recent studies suggest that degeneration of the serotonergic pathway also contributes to depression and apathy. A meta-analysis revealed that 57.2% of apathetic PD patients suffer from depression, while the remaining 42.8% experience apathy as a symptom distinct from depression [56]. The severity of apathy is primarily associated with specific lesions in the caudate nucleus and orbitofrontal cortex, whereas depression is linked to the anterior cingulate cortex. These distinct neural correlates may explain the differences in these symptoms [57]. Thus, cholinergic inhibitors can relieve apathy by increasing cholinergic neurotransmission but do not interfere with depressive symptoms. These results indicate that dopaminergic pathways may involve both apathy and depression, while serotonergic pathways may involve these symptoms in different ways [58].

In the case of anxiety combined with depression in PD, which is also frequent, the degree of both depression and anxiety is linked to changes in the serotonergic pathway, as well as the loss of dopamine and norepinephrine innervation, confirming the relationship of dopaminergic, serotonergic, and noradrenergic pathways in the dynamics of both pathologies [58].

4. The neurophysiology of Parkinson's disease

Neurophysiology consists of another branch of neuroscience, characterized as behavioral neuroscience, that is, the relationship of the nervous system with human behavior. It includes the study of functions such as sleep, gait, coordination, and sensory responses, among others [59]. One of the ways we can obtain physiological information is through the electroencephalogram (EEG), a technique that captures the postsynaptic electrical activity of the cerebral cortex *via* electrodes and transforms it into brain waves.

In general, the electrodes capture the electrical responses of layers III and V, formed by pyramidal cells in the cortex, which occur near the scalp. These responses are characterized by the postsynaptic potential difference of billions of neurons in the area near the electrode [60]. The potential difference forms a two-dimensional topographic representation of cortical activity that can then be mathematically processed through the Fourier transform. Thus, the Fourier transform is a way of decomposing the sinusoidal signals captured by cortical depolarization. Generally, there are two EEG patterns in wakeful states: the first is marked by synchronization, that is, rhythmic activity of high amplitude and low frequency, usually measured with eyes closed. The second is desynchronized activity, which is irregular, of low amplitude or voltage, and high frequency, occurring during visual attention with eyes open. EEG synchronization is recorded in the alpha frequency range (8–11 Hz) and results from thalamic oscillations whose cells fire rhythmically, with an inhibitory function, while desynchronized activity corresponds to increased cortical activity generated by sensory inputs, at which time cortical and thalamic neurons fire in tonic mode [61].

In general, cortical activity recorded by electrodes can be categorized into the following frequency bands: delta: 1–4 Hz, theta: 4–8 Hz, alpha: 8–13 Hz, beta: 13–30 Hz, and gamma: 30–60 Hz.

The frequency is inversely proportional to the wave amplitude, which means that when the frequency is high, the amplitude is low, and when the frequency is low, the amplitude is high [62]. There are some associations between frequency bands, cortical activity, and behaviors performed, that is, when there is intense cortical activity, faster waves are involved in certain brain areas, and some behavior is associated with the activity. Thus, schematically and simply, there are associations between delta waves, which are low-frequency cortical activity, with deep sleep; theta and alpha waves, with moderate and low cortical activity, related to working memory, attention, and creativity; beta and gamma waves, are associated with intense thought activity, such as stimulus integration [63], and beta waves are also associated with cortical desynchronization observed during wakefulness and REM sleep [59].

Regarding the neurophysiology of PD, beta oscillations play an important role in movement coordination. They are predominant during stability, tonic contractions, decreasing immediately before and during movement execution, with a rebound shortly after [64].

Studies support the idea that stopping or omitting undesirable behaviors is associated with increased synchronization and coherence of beta frequency oscillations [65]. Thus, in Parkinson's cases, alteration of beta frequency oscillations in the dorsolateral and frontal regions can be observed, which may be related to motor processing, specifically in stopping movement. Striatal dopaminergic denervation leads to excessive beta oscillatory synchronization with the thalamo-cortical circuits and basal nuclei. Coherence at 15–30 Hz in the somatosensory area produces symptom relief in Parkinson's disease [66].

Animal models and electrophysiological studies for PD linked dopaminergic denervation to excessive beta synchronization with basal and thalamo-cortical circuits. For example, two studies demonstrated that treatment with L-dopa reduced coherence in beta frequencies between the GPi and the subthalamic nucleus (STN), and between the STN and the supplementary motor area (SMA) during rest or motor tasks [67, 68].

Interhemispheric beta synchronization may be another electrophysiological feature of PD [6]. Additionally, Parkinson's patients who underwent DBS implant surgery have shown beta oscillations in the dorsolateral region, topographically associated with motor areas [69]. In this context, it is believed that beta band synchronization represents a rhythm that promoting immutability, stabilizing the neural circuit in a state of low entropy and maintaining homeostasis [70]. The greater the beta oscillatory synchronization, the larger the neural circuits can encompass distant regions in predictable and stereotyped spatiotemporal firing patterns. Thus, notably, excessive beta synchronization is potentially related to symptoms of bradykinesia and rigidity [71], as beta synchronization facilitates the stopping behavior through the direct and indirect pathways of the *substantia nigra pars compacta* and the *putamen* [72], while oscillations may explain tremor and dyskinesia, respectively [73].

The gamma frequency (35–90 hz) plays a fundamental role in neuronal computation, being the consequence of inhibitory postsynaptic potential, reverberating in interneural networks, and between inhibitory and excitatory neurons of pyramidal populations, causing a recurrent feedback loop [74, 75]. Additionally, it is associated with motor processing, and its excessive synchronization can potentially lead to chaotic kinesthetic activity characterizing dyskinesia syndromes.

Matzilevich et al. [76] suggest that the interaction between beta and gamma oscillations may represent a coupling mechanism that subserves the maintenance of motor programming and task mediation. For example, exaggerated coupling between the low-frequency beta band phase (13–22 Hz) and the high-frequency gamma band amplitude (300 Hz) within the STN is correlated with bradykinesia and rigidity severity [77].

Furthermore, regarding alpha waves, DBS reduces the amplitude of this frequency band over the sensorimotor cortex. This aligns with the notion that the basal ganglia promote alpha desynchronization by releasing motor regions from an idle state, thereby facilitating the effective selection and programming of motor responses [76].

Excessive theta oscillation coincides with the resting tremor frequency in Parkinsonism and may represent an underlying mechanism for this symptom [6]. Theta oscillations are also associated with gait disturbances in PD, with increased frontal theta oscillations seemingly related to the transition to gait freezing, possibly reflecting a compensatory cognitive mechanism. Conversely, decreased theta oscillations in the occipital region are linked to gait imbalance [76].

5. The use of neurofeedback in Parkinson's disease

Neurofeedback (NFB) is a form of neuromodulation through operant conditioning of brain activity, where a computational interface provides visual and/or auditory feedback to the subject as they achieve the expected results [78].

Neurofeedback can use cortical information captured by electroencephalogram (EEG) or functional near-infrared spectrography (fNIRS) [79], as well as deep brain information captured by functional magnetic resonance imaging (fMRI) [80].

The principle governing neurofeedback is operant conditioning, in which a computational interface provides visual and/or auditory feedback to the subject as they achieve the expected results [81]. However, according to Lacroix's cognitive proposal (1986), the subject also consciously appropriates their physiological responses by perceiving the change in mental state, making NFB also governed by cognitive principles [82].

As a form of neuromodulation, NFB training promotes the persistent functional reorganization of the brain through neuroplasticity, evidenced by cortical changes observed post-training. These changes are based on Hebbian cellular learning principles [81].

The most common form of neurofeedback is through EEG, where brain waves are the neurophysiological aspect being trained. EEG neurofeedback is the most widely used type of neuromodulation biofeedback due to its easy handling, adaptability to everyday life, and having more systematic and proven protocols [78]. EEG NFB is based on operant conditioning of brain waves according to frequency bands associated with certain physiological aspects. Additionally, its action on the brain is dynamic, meaning a particular frequency band can be increased in a specific region while decreasing in another to achieve a result [83].

Generally, electrodes are installed in the target region of the scalp associated with a cortical area, and the computational interface will provide feedback to the subject when they reach the established frequency band associated with the desired modification. For example, the protocol used to improve attention deficit hyperactivity disorder (ADHD) [84–86] is performed in the central cortex region, where the electrode is placed at Cz, and the training frequency band is the increase of the sensorimotor rhythm (SMR), with a frequency of 12–15 Hz. Thus, when the individual increases the SMR in this region, there is computational feedback to reinforce the behavior, and the consequent sensation of improved attention also helps the individual to self-regulate.

Neurofeedback has various protocols besides the example cited above and can be applied to several clinical conditions such as epilepsy [87], anxiety [88], and depression [89] in extensively studied protocols, both in the central cortex region to increase SMR (12–15 Hz) and in the frontal cortex region [81]. The sensorimotor rhythm occurs more precisely over the primary motor cortex and was first observed during the operant conditioning of cats alongside the analysis of cortical activity. The conditioning involved training to receive food when the animals pressed a bar, and when the cats waited for the food after pressing the bar, a decrease in movement and an increase in alertness associated with activation in the 12–15 Hz range was observed [90]. In humans, the SMR follows a similar pattern [91], meaning that an increase in 12–15 Hz activity in the sensorimotor area corresponds to a suppression of movement and an enhancement of attention.

Regarding motor symptoms improvement in Parkinson's disease, a review conducted by Anil et al. [13] on experimental articles using all forms of neurofeedback to enhance motor function in PD patients demonstrated that most of them applied the alpha/beta rhythm protocol similarly to the protocol used for ADHD, where SMR training occurs in the sensorimotor region since the circuits involved in SMR action are thalamocortical networks that reduce interference from somatosensory information conduction. This inhibition caused by the SMR increase leads to better integration of information processing in the cortex, as motor activity can interfere with this processing, hindering cognitive performance [92]. Thus, SMR NF training acts on the inhibitory mechanisms of thalamic circuits [93].

Additionally, beta synchronization changes in the motor region are predominant in individuals with PD, as mentioned earlier. Apparently, NF results with fMRI are more promising than with EEG, but it should be considered that using MRI implies a hospital context, is restrictive, and demands a high cost, whereas EEG would have broader applicability, being portable and potentially usable outside the clinical context [94].

NFB can be an alternative for controlling motor symptoms in PD patients since the SMR protocol in the sensorimotor region, besides affecting attention, can also inhibit the hyperactivity characteristic of ADHD patients, as increasing this rhythm involves regulating high motor command [95].

The study conducted by Shi et al. [96] tested the effect of multimodal biofeedback (BFB) on motor and non-motor symptoms in PD, comparing a sample divided into three groups: placebo, EEG NFB, and multimodal BFB. The multimodal group performed the SMR training protocol at C3 and C4, heartbeat through electrocardiogram, and blood oxygenation; the NFB group did only the SMR protocol, and the placebo group did a false NFB.

The results showed that multimodal BFB improved non-motor symptoms, specifically depression, due to neuromodulation of the parietal and frontal lobes, especially in theta waves. Additionally, NFB training improved motor symptoms, mainly by regulating beta waves [96].

Another study applied the SMR protocol to a PD patient [97], as this brain activity over the sensorimotor cortex is associated with motor planning, initiation, and imagination [98]. Thus, they tested a single case using fMRI neurofeedback (NFB) in the ON and OFF dopaminergic medication states to check the feasibility of NFB training for this purpose, as motor imagination training in fMRI NFB has shown to induce improvement in motor function in PD patients [99]. The results were mixed on motor behavior, and cortical analysis showed that beta activity reduced at the end of the patient's training in the ON medication state.

Furthermore, SMR strength was initially distributed over the posterior region and, by the end of the training, was more centralized over the motor cortex. Changes in the spatial distribution of theta and alpha suggest that the patient might be learning cognitive control strategies [97]. This could indicate that theta oscillations in the medial frontal region are integrating the training information [100, 101].

Moreover, according to Gomez et al. [102], SMR provides an event-related desynchronization (ERD) in beta activity and a rebound in event-related synchronization in alpha (ERS), which might lead to long-term potentiation and, consequently, brain plasticity [103].

An important aspect to mention is that NFB in the elderly population is a tendency for the formation of cognitive reserve, as published works have demonstrated the enhancement of cognitive performance in terms of attention, memory, and working memory through protocols to increase alpha peak [104], suppress theta [105], increase theta [106], increase theta and alpha [107, 108], and increase SMR [109, 110].

The proposal to use NFB for elderly individuals presenting mild cognitive impairment or dementia was reviewed by Trambraiolli et al. [111]. The authors demonstrated that studies are scarce and have varied protocols, but their results indicate improvement in memory and working memory, and they also demonstrate that it is a promising form of treatment for individuals with affected cognitive capacity.

Besides cognitive decline and neuropsychiatric alterations observed in Parkinson's disease patients, they also present sensorimotor difficulties, which impair the integration between attention and action, potentially interfering with these individuals' emotional and cognitive aspects [112].

Thus, NFB might be a tool to provide cognitive reserve in individuals with PD as well as to regulate neuropsychiatric symptoms, being applied not only to improve motor function but rather to provide quality of life-changing their non-motor symptoms.

6. Conclusion

To conclude, the main purpose of the chapter was to enlighten people about the use of NFB as a tool for PD in many aspects of its symptoms. PD is a degenerative disease of the central nervous system and implies many impairments to patients as it progresses; not only do motor symptoms harm daily living activities but also non-motor symptoms impact the quality of life and social skills of those individuals.

As a neurodegenerative disease the alterations of neurophysiology in PD are inevitable; however, as NFB may provide plasticity, this training might be able to supply brain reserve and favor the delay of its progression.

Moreover, as cognitive performance is an important issue for social skills and individual executive function, as well as emotional regulation also plays an important role in personal life, NFB also may provide cognitive reserve and emotional regulation, maintaining the quality of life and regular activities for those individuals.

Therefore, it was presented some of the studies that have tested NFB protocols to improve motor and non-motor function in PD patients, with results indicating that it might improve motor function generally and depressive symptoms, as well as cognitive protocols to general cognitive decline in the elderly, have pointed to an improvement in attention, memory, and working memory.

Acknowledgements

We thank the laboratory psychology interns Luisa Wakim Batista and Patricia Cardoso da Silva for assistance in collecting the data and the Laboratory of Neuroscience and Behavior, University of Brasília, Brazil.

Conflicts of interest

The authors declare no conflict of interest.

Author details

Valeska Kouzak*, Maria Clotilde Tavares and Wendy Isabel Silvestre da Silva
University of Brasília, Brasília, Brazil

*Address all correspondence to: valeskakouzak@gmail.com

References

[1] Tysnes OB, Storstein A. Epidemiology of Parkinson's disease. Journal of Neural Transmission. 2017;**124**:901-905. DOI: 10.1007/s00702-017-1686-y

[2] Dorsey ER, Elbaz A. Global, regional, and national burden of Parkinson's disease, 1990-2016: A systematic analysis for the global burden of disease study 2016. The Lancet Neurology. 2018;**17**(11):939-953

[3] Abbas MM, Xu Z, Tan LC. Epidemiology of Parkinson's disease—East versus west. Movement Disorders Clinical Practice. 2018;**5**:14-28. DOI: 10.1002/mdc3.12568

[4] Simon DK, Tanner CM, Brundin P. Parkinson disease epidemiology, pathology, genetics, and pathophysiology. Clinics in Geriatric Medicine. 2020;**36**(1):1-12. DOI: 10.1016/j.cger.2019.08.002

[5] Brandão PRP et al. Cognitive impairment in Parkinson's disease: A clinical and pathophysiological overview. Journal of the Neurological Sciences. 2020;**419**:117177. DOI: 10.1016/j.jns.2020.117177

[6] Esmail S, Linden DE. Neural networks and neurofeedback in Parkinson's disease. NeuroRegulation. 2014;**1**(3-4):240-272. DOI: 10.15540/nr.1.3-4.240

[7] Braak H et al. Stages in the development of Parkinson's disease-related pathology. Cell and Tissue Research. 2004;**318**(1):121-134. DOI: 10.1007/s00441-004-0956-9

[8] Paredes-Rodriguez E, Vegas-Suarez S, Morera-Herreras T, De Deurwaerdere P, Miguelez C. The noradrenergic system in Parkinson's disease. Frontiers in Pharmacology. 2020;**11**:435

[9] Paulus W, Jellinger K. The neuropathologic basis of different clinical subgroups of Parkinson's disease. Journal of Neuropathology and Experimental Neurology. 1991;**50**(6):743-755. DOI: 10.1097/00005072-199111000-00006

[10] Jellinger KA, Paulus W. Clinico-pathological correlations in Parkinson's disease. Clinical Neurology and Neurosurgery. 1992;**94**:86-88

[11] Albin RL, Young AB, Penney JB. The functional anatomy of basal ganglia disorders. Trends in Neurosciences. 1989;**12**:366-375

[12] Hartmann CJ, Fliegen S, Groiss SJ, Wojtecki L, Schnitzler A. An update on best practice of deep brain stimulation in Parkinson's disease. Therapeutic Advances in Neurologic Disorders. 2019;**12**:1-20. DOI: 10.1177/1756286419838096

[13] Anil K, Hall SD, Demain S, Freeman JA, Ganis G, Marsden J. A systematic review of neurofeedback for the management of motor symptoms in Parkinson's disease. Brain Sciences. 2021;**11**(10):1292. DOI: 10.3390/brainsci11101292

[14] Schlesinger I, Sinai A, Zaaroor M. MRI-Guided Focused Ultrasound in Parkinson's Disease: A Review. Parkinson's Disease. 2017;**2017**(1):8124624. DOI: 10.1155/2017/8124624

[15] Luria AR. The Working Memory. Basic Books—A Member of the Perseus. Reino Unido: Book Company; 1973

[16] Gazzaniga MS, Ivry RB, Mangun GR. Cognitive Neuroscience—The Biology of the Mind. 4th ed. New York: W.W. Norton; 2014

[17] Piccinini G. Neurocognitive Mechanisms: Explaining Biological Cognition. Oxford, UK: Oxford University Press; 2020

[18] Jenner et al. Parkinson's disease—The debate on the clinical phenomenology, aetiology, pathology and pathogenesis. Journal of Parkinson's Disease. 2013;**3**: 1-11. DOI: 10.3233/JPD-13017

[19] Brandão PRDP. Comprometimento cognitivo na doença de Parkinson: Correlatos clínicos, neuropsicológicos e de neuroimagem. Brasil, Brasília: UnB; 2022

[20] Aarsland D et al. Mild cognitive impairment in Parkinson disease: A multicenter pooled analysis. Neurology. 2010;**75**(12):1062-1069. DOI: 10.1212/WNL.0b013e3181f39d0e

[21] Papagno C, Trojano L. Cognitive and behavioral disorders in Parkinson's disease: An update. I: Cognitive impairments. Neurological Sciences. 2018;**39**(2):215-223

[22] Kehagia AA, Barker RA, Robbins TW. Cognitive impairment in Parkinson's disease: The dual syndrome hypothesis. Neurodegenerative Diseases. 2013;**11**(2):79-92. DOI: 10.1159/000341998

[23] Barvas E, Mattavelli G, Zappini F, Giardina F, Ottaviani D, Papagno C. Cognitive phenotypes in Parkinson's disease: A latent profile analysis. Neuropsychology. 2021;**35**(4):451

[24] Loftus AM, Gasson N, Lopez N, Sellner M, Reid C, Cocks N, et al. Cognitive reserve, executive function, and memory in Parkinson's disease. Brain Sciences. 2021;**11**(8):992

[25] Beyer MK, Aarsland D. Grey matter atrophy in early versus late dementia in Parkinson's disease. Parkinsonism and Related Disorders. 2008;**14**(8):620-625. DOI: 10.1016/j.parkreldis.2008.01.021

[26] Kenny ER, Burton EJ, O'Brien JT. A volumetric magnetic resonance imaging study of entorhinal cortex volume in dementia with lewy bodies. A comparison with Alzheimer's disease and Parkinson's disease with and without dementia. Dementia and Geriatric Cognitive Disorders. 2008;**26**(3):218-225. DOI: 10.1159/000153432

[27] Laakso MP et al. Hippocampal volumes in Alzheimer's disease, Parkinson's disease with and without dementia, and in vascular dementia: An MRI study. Neurology. 1996;**46**(3):678-681. DOI: 10.1212/wnl.46.3.678

[28] Ellfolk U et al. Brain volumetric correlates of memory in early Parkinson's disease. Journal of Parkinson's Disease. 2013;**3**(4):593-601. DOI: 10.3233/JPD-130276

[29] Pereira JB, Hall S, Jalakas M, Grothe MJ, Strandberg O, Stomrud E, et al. Longitudinal degeneration of the basal forebrain predicts subsequent dementia in Parkinson's disease. Neurobiology of Disease. 2020;**139**:104831

[30] Pereira JB et al. Assessment of cortical degeneration in patients with Parkinson's disease by voxel-based morphometry, cortical folding, and cortical thickness. Human Brain Mapping. 2012;**33**(11):2521-2534. DOI: 10.1002/hbm.21378

[31] Pereira JB et al. Neuroanatomical substrate of visuospatial and

visuoperceptual impairment in Parkinson's disease. Movement Disorders. 2009;**24**(8):1193-1199. DOI: 10.1002/mds.22560

[32] Koh SB et al. Stereopsis and extrastriate cortical atrophy in Parkinson's disease: A voxel-based morphometric study. Neuroreport. 2013;**24**(5):229-232. DOI: 10.1097/WNR.0b013e32835edbc5

[33] Pereira JB et al. Cortical thinning in patients with REM sleep behavior disorder is associated with clinical progression. NPJ Parkinsons Disease. 2019;**5**:7. DOI: 10.1038/s41531-019-0079-3

[34] Pereira JB et al. Initial cognitive decline is associated with cortical thinning in early Parkinson disease. Neurology. 2014;**82**(22):2017-2025. DOI: 10.1212/WNL.0000000000000483

[35] Goldman JG et al. Corpus callosal atrophy and associations with cognitive impairment in Parkinson disease. Neurology. 2017;**88**(13):1265-1272. DOI: 10.1212/WNL.0000000000003764

[36] Mak E et al. Longitudinal whole-brain atrophy and ventricular enlargement in nondemented Parkinson's disease. Neurobiology of Aging. 2017;**55**:78-90. DOI: 10.1016/j.neurobiolaging.2017.03.012

[37] Brandão PRP, Pereira DA, Grippe TC, Bispo DDC, Maluf FB, Yunes MP, et al. Parkinson's disease-cognitive rating scale (PD-CRS): Normative data and mild cognitive impairment assessment in Brazil. Movements Disorder Clinical Practice. 2023;**10**(3):452-465. DOI: 10.1002/mdc3.13657

[38] Seppi K, Ray Chaudhuri K, Coelho M, Fox SH, Katzenschlager R, Perez Lloret S, et al. Update on treatments for nonmotor symptoms of Parkinson's disease-an evidence-based medicine review. Movement Disorders. 2019;**34**:180-198. DOI: 10.1002/mds.27602

[39] Aarsland D, Marsh L, Schrag A. Neuropsychiatric symptoms in Parkinson's disease. Movement Disorders: Official Journey of the Movement Disorder. 2009;**24**(15):2175-2186. DOI: 10.1002/mds.22589

[40] Postuma RB et al. MDS clinical diagnostic criteria for Parkinson's disease. Movement Disorders. 2015;**30**(12):1591-1601. DOI: 10.1002/mds.26424

[41] Kalia LV, Lang AE. Parkinson's disease. Lancet. 2015;**386**(9996):896-912. DOI: 10.1016/S0140-6736(14)61393-3

[42] De Micco R, Satolli S, Siciliano M, Di Nardo F, Caiazzo G, Russo A, et al. Connectivity correlates of anxiety symptoms in drug-naive Parkinson's disease patients. Movement Disorders. 2021;**36**(1):96-105

[43] Carey G, Lopes R, Moonen AJ, Mulders AE, de Jong JJ, Kuchcinski G, et al. Cognitive behavioral therapy for anxiety in Parkinson's disease induces functional brain changes. Journal of Parkinson's Disease. 2023;**13**(1):93-103

[44] Garlovsky JK, Overton PG, Simpson J. Psychological predictors of anxiety and depression in Parkinson's disease: A systematic review. Journal of Clinical Psychology. 2016;**72**(10):979-998

[45] Carey G, Gormezo M, Jong de JJA, Hofman PAM, Backes WH, Dujardin K, et al. Neuroimaging of anxiety in Parkinson's disease: A systematic review. Movement Disorders. 2020;**36**:327-339

[46] Péron J, Dondaine T, Le Jeune F, Grandjean D, Vérin M. Emotional processing in Parkinson's disease: A systematic review. Movement Disorders. 2012;**27**(2):186-199

[47] Chen CPLH, Alder JT, Bray L, Kingsbury AE, Francis PT, Foster OJF. Post-synaptic 5-HT1a and 5-HT2a receptors are increased in Parkinson's disease neocortex. Annals of the New York Academy of Sciences. 1998;**861**:288-289

[48] Leentjens AF, Scholtissen B, Vreeling FW, Verhey FR. The serotonergic hypothesis for depression in Parkinson's disease: An experimental approach. Neuropsychopharmacology. 2006;**31**(5):1009-1015

[49] Benarroch EE. Serotonergic modulation of basal ganglia circuits: Complexity and therapeutic opportunities. Neurology. 2009;**73**(11):880-886

[50] Leentjens AF, Dujardin K, Marsh L, Martinez-Martin P, Richard IH, Starkstein SE, et al. Anxiety rating scales in Parkinson's disease: Critique and recommendations. Movement Disorders: Official Journal of the Movement Disorder Society. 2008;**23**(14):2015-2025

[51] Aarsland D et al. Cognitive impairment in incident, untreated Parkinson disease: The Norwegian Park West study. Neurology. 2009;**72**(13):1121-1126. DOI: 10.1212/01.wnl.0000338632.00552.cb

[52] Galts CP, Bettio LE, Jewett DC, Yang CC, Brocardo PS, Rodrigues ALS, et al. Depression in neurodegenerative diseases: Common mechanisms and current treatment options. Neuroscience and Biobehavioral Reviews. 2019;**102**:56-84

[53] Jankovic J, Tan EK. Parkinson's disease: Etiopathogenesis and treatment. Journal of Neurology, Neurosurgery and Psychiatry. 2020;**91**(8):795-808

[54] Mueller C, Rajkumar AP, Wan YM, Velayudhan L, Ffytche D, Chaudhuri KR, et al. Assessment and management of neuropsychiatric symptoms in Parkinson's disease. CNS Drugs. 2018;**32**(7):621-635

[55] Castrioto A, Thobois S, Anheim M, Quesada JL, Lhommée E, Klinger H, et al. A randomized controlled double-blind study of rotigotine on neuropsychiatric symptoms in de novo PD. NPJ Parkinson's Disease. 2020;**6**(1):41

[56] Devos D, Moreau C, Maltête D, Lefaucheur R, Kreisler A, Eusebio A, et al. Rivastigmine in apathetic but dementia and depression-free patients with Parkinson's disease: A double-blind, placebo-controlled, randomised clinical trial. Journal of Neurology, Neurosurgery and Psychiatry. 2014;**85**(6):668-674

[57] Maillet A, Krack P, Lhommée E, Météreau E, Klinger H, Favre E, et al. The prominent role of serotonergic degeneration in apathy, anxiety and depression in de novo Parkinson's disease. Brain. 2016;**139**(9):2486-2502

[58] Cong S, Xiang C, Zhang S, Zhang T, Wang H, Cong S. Prevalence and clinical aspects of depression in Parkinson's disease: A systematic review and meta-analysis of 129 studies. 2022. DOI: 10.1016/j.neubiorev.2022.104749

[59] Lent R. Cem bilhões de neurônios. Conceitos fundamentais de neurociência. 2010;**2**:631-639

[60] Teplan M. Fundamentals of EEG measurement. Measurement Science Review. 2002;**2**(2):1-11

[61] Neumann NICOLA, Strehl U, Birbaumer NIELS. A primer of electroencephalographic instrumentation. In: Biofeedback: A practitioner's Guide. 2003. pp. 88-102

[62] Kaiser DA. Basic principles of quantitative EEG. Journal of Adult Development. 2005;**12**(2/3):99-104

[63] Demos JN. Getting Started with Neurofeedback. New York, NY: W.W. Norton and Company; 2005

[64] Alegre M, Lopez-Azcarate J, Obeso I, Wilkinson L, Rodriguez-Oroz MC, Valencia M, et al. The subthalamic nucleus is involved in successful inhibition in the stop-signal task: A local field potential study in Parkinson's disease. Experimental Neurology. 2013;**239**:1-12. DOI: 10.1016/j.expneurol.2012.08.027

[65] Gilbertson T, Lalo E, Doyle L, Di Lazzaro V, Cioni B, Brown P. Existing motor state is favored at the expense of new movement during 13-35 Hz oscillatory synchrony in the human corticospinal system. Journal of Neuroscience. 2005;**25**:7771-7779

[66] Marsden JF, Limousin-Dowsey P, Ashby P, Pollak P, Brown P. Subthalamic nucleus, sensorimotor cortex and muscle interrelationships in Parkinson's disease. Brain. 2001;**124**:378-388

[67] Brown P, Oliviero A, Mazzone P, et al. Dopamine dependency of oscillations between subthalamic nucleus and pallidum in Parkinson's disease. The Journal of Neuroscience. 2001;**21**(3):1033-1038

[68] Cassidy M, Mazzone P, Oliviero A, et al. Movement-related changes in synchronization in the human basal ganglia. Brain. 2002;**125**(6):1235-1246

[69] Romanelli P, Esposito V, Schaal DW, Heit G. Somatotopy in the basal ganglia: Experimental and clinical evidence for segregated sensorimotor channels. Brain Research Reviews. 2005;**48**:112-128

[70] Engel AK, Fries P. Beta-band oscillations—Signalling the status quo? Current Opinion in Neurobiology. 2010;**20**:156-165. DOI: 10.1016/j.conb.2010.02.015

[71] Zaidel A, Spivak A, Grieb B, Bergman H, Israel Z. Subthalamic span of β oscillations predicts deep brain stimulation efficacy for patients with Parkinson's disease. Brain. 2010;**133**(7):2007-2021

[72] Mehler DMA. Turning markers into targets—Scoping neural circuits for motor neurofeedback training in Parkinson's disease. Brain-Apparatus Communication: A Journal of Bacomics. 2022;**1**(1):1-27. DOI: 10.1080/27706710.2022.2061300

[73] Richter U, Halje P, Petersson P. Mechanisms underlying cortical resonant states: Implications for levodopa-induced dyskinesia. Reviews in the Neurosciences. 2013;**24**:415-429. DOI: 10.1515/revneuro-2013-0018

[74] Fries P. Neuronal gamma-band synchronization as a fundamental process in cortical computation. Annual Review of Neuroscience. 2009;**32**:209-224. DOI: 10.1146/annurev.neuro.051508.135603

[75] Buzsáki G, Wang XJ. Mechanisms of gamma oscillations. Annual Review of Neuroscience. 2012;**35**:203-225. DOI: 10.1146/annurev-neuro-062111-150444

[76] Matzilevich EU, Daniel PL, Little S. Towards therapeutic electrophysiological

neurofeedback in Parkinson's disease. Parkinsonism and Related Disorders. 2024;**106010**

[77] van Wijk BC, Beudel M, Jha A, Oswal A, Foltynie T, Hariz MI, et al. Subthalamic nucleus phase–amplitude coupling correlates with motor impairment in Parkinson's disease. Clinical Neurophysiology. 2016;**127**(4):2010-2019

[78] Kouzak V. Neurociências para idosos: treino da memória operacional por meio do neurofeedback. Belo Horizonte, MG-Brasil: Editora Dialética; 2020

[79] Kober SE, Wood G. Changes in hemodynamic signals accompanying motor imagery and motor execution of swallowing: A near-infrared spectroscopy study. NeuroImage. 2014;**93**:1-10

[80] Soares JM, Magalhães R, Moreira PS, Sousa A, Ganz E, Sampaio A, et al. Hitchhiker's guide to functional magnetic resonance. Frontiers in Neuroscience. 2016;**10**

[81] Sitaram R, Ros T, Stoeckel L, Haller S, Scharnowski F, Lewis-Peacock J, et al. Closed-loop brain training: The science of neurofeedback. Nature Reviews. Neuroscience. 2017;**18**:86-100. DOI: 10.1038/nrn.2016.164

[82] Strehl U. What learning theories can teach us in designing neurofeedback treatments. Frontiers in Human Neuroscience. 2014;**8**(894):1-8

[83] Paz VKC, Tomaz C. Neurofeedback training on aging: Prospects on maintaining cognitive reserve. In: Shad KF, Dogan KH, editors. Neurological and Mental Disorders. London, UK: IntechOpen. Available from: https://www.intechopen.com/chapters/70786; 2020. DOI: 10.5772/intechopen.90847

[84] Thompson M, Thompson L. The Neurofeedback Book-An Introduction to Basic Concepts in Applied Psychophysiology. Colorado, EUA: The Applied Psychophysiology and Biofeedback; 2003

[85] Monastra VJ, Lynn S, Linden M, Lubar JF, Gruzilier J, LaVaque TJ. Electroencephalographic biofeedback in the treatment of attention deficit/hyperactivity disorder. Applied Psychophysiology and Biofeedback. 2005;**30**:95-114. DOI: 10.1007/s10484-005-4305-x

[86] Vernon D, Egner T, Cooper N, Compton T, Neilands C, Sheri A, et al. The effect of training distinct neurofeedback protocols on aspects of cognitive performance. International Journal of Psychophysiology. 2003;**47**(1):75-85

[87] Sterman MB. Physiological origins and functional correlates of EEG rhythmic activities: Implications for self-regulation. Biofeedback Self Regul. 1996;**21**:3-33. DOI: 10.1007/bf02214147

[88] Hammond D. Neurofeedback training for anxiety and depression. Journal of Adult Development. 2005;**12**:131-137. DOI: 10.1007/s10804-005-7029-5

[89] Esmail S, Linden DEJ. Emotion regulation networks and neurofeedback in depression. Cognitive Sciences. 2011;**6**(2):101-128

[90] Sterman MB, Howe RC, Macdonald LR. Facilitation of spindle-burst sleep by conditioning of electroencephalographic activity while awake. Science. 1970;**167**(3921):1146-1148

[91] Sterman MB. Basic concepts and clinical findings in the treatment of seisures. 2000

[92] Kober SE, Witte M, Stangl M, Väljamäe A, Neuper C, Wood G. Shutting down sensorimotor interference unblocks the networks for stimulus processing: An SMR neurofeedback training study. Clinical Neurophysiology. 2015;**126**:82-95. DOI: 10.1016/j.clinph.2014.03.031

[93] Egner T, Gruzelier J. EEG biofeedback of low b band components: Frequency specific effects on variables of attention and event- related brain potentials. Clinical Neurophysiology. 2004;**115**:131-139. DOI: 10.1016/s1388-2457(03)00353-5

[94] Sherwood MS, Kane JH, Weisend MP, Parker JG. Enhanced control of dorsolateral prefrontal cortex neurophysiology with real-time functional magnetic resonance imaging (rt-fMRI) neurofeedback training and working memory practice. NeuroImage. 2016;**124**:214-223

[95] Witte M, Kober SE, Ninaus M, Neuper C, Wood G. Control beliefs can predict the ability to up-regulate sensorimotor rhythm during neurofeedback training. Frontiers in Human Neuroscience. 2013;**7**:478

[96] Shi Z, Ding L, Han X, Jiang B, Zhang J, Suo D, et al. Multimodal biofeedback for Parkinson's disease motor and nonmotor symptoms. Brain Science Advances. 2023;**9**(2):136-154

[97] Cook AJ, Pfeifer KJ, Tass PA. A single case feasibility study of sensorimotor rhythm neurofeedback in Parkinson's disease. Frontiers in Neuroscience. 2021;**15**:623317

[98] Stefano, Filho CA, Attux R, Castellano G. Motor imagery neurofeedback: From system conceptualization to neural correlates. Current Behavioral Neuroscience Reports. 2024;**11**:78-98

[99] Tinaz S, Kamel S, Aravala SS, Elfil M, Aayoumi A, Patel A, et al. Neurofeedback-guided kinesthetic motor imagery training in Parkinson's disease: Randomized trial. NeuroImage: Clinical. 2022;(34). DOI: 10.1016/j.nicl.2022.102980

[100] Cavanagh JF, Frank MJ. Frontal theta as a mechanism for cognitive control. Trends in Cognitive Sciences. 2014;**18**:414-421. DOI: 10.1016/j.tics.2014.04.012

[101] Luft CD. Learning from feedback: The neural mechanisms of feedback processing facilitating better performance. Behavioural Brain Research. 2014;**261**:356-336

[102] Gomez-Pilar J, Corralejo R, Nicolas-Alonso LF, Álvarez D, Hornero R. Neurofeedback training with a motor imagery-based BCI: Neurocognitive improvements and EEG changes in the elderly. Medical and Biological Engineering and Computing. 2016;**54**:1655-1666

[103] Ros T, Munneke MAM, Parkinson LA, Gruzelier JH. Neurofeedback facilitation of implicit motor learning. Biological Psychology. 2014;**95**:54-58

[104] Angelakis E, Stathopoulou S, Frymiare JL, Green DL, Lubar JF, Kounios J. EEG neurofeedback: A brief overview and an example of peak alpha frequency training for cognitive enhancement in the elderly. The Clinical Neuropsychologist. 2007;**21**(1):110-129

[105] Becerra J, Fernandez T, Roca-Stappung M, Diaz-Comas L,

Galán L, Bosch J, et al Neurofeedback in healthy elderly human subjects with electroencephalographic risk for cognitive disorder. Journal of Alzheimer's Disease. 2012;**28**(2):357-367

[106] Juhel J. The effects of neurofeedback training on memory performance in elderly subjects. Psychology. 2011;**2**(08):846

[107] Wang JR, Hsieh S. Neurofeedback training improves working memory and attention performance. Clinical Neurophysiology. 2013;**124**(12)

[108] Reis J, Portugal AM, Fernandes L, Afonso N, Pereira M, Sousa N, et al. An alpha and theta intensive and short neurofeedback protocol for healthy aging working memory training. Frontiers in Aging Neuroscience. 2016;**8**:1-11

[109] Campos da Paz VK, Garcia A, da Paz C, Neto A, Tomaz C. SMR neurofeedback facilitates working memory performance in healthy older adults: A behavior and EEG study. Frontiers in Behavioral Neuroscience. 2018;**12**:1-11. DOI: 10.3389/fnbeh.2018.00321

[110] Marlats F, Bao G, Chevallier S, Boubaya M, Djabelkhir-Jemmi L, Wu YH, et al. SMR/theta neurofeedback training improves cognitive performance and EEG activity in elderly with mild cognitive impairment: A pilot study. Frontiers in Aging Neuroscience. 2020;**12**(147):1-11. DOI: 10.3389/fnagi.2020.00147

[111] Trambraiolli LR, Cassani R, Mehler DN, Falk T. Neurofeedback and the aging brain: A systematic review of training protocols for dementia and mild cognitive impairment. Frontiers in Aging Neuroscience. 2021;**13**. DOI: 10.3389/fnagi.2021.682683

[112] Saito N, Takahata K, Yamakado H, et al. Altered awareness of action in Parkinson's disease: Evaluations by explicit and implicit measures. Scientific Reports. 2017;7:8019. DOI: 10.1038/s41598-017-08482-0